THE DIABETES

weight-loss

COOKBOOK

A life-changing diet
to prevent and reverse
type 2 diabetes

KATIE *&* **GIANCARLO CALDESI**

WITH JENNY PHILLIPS

Photography by Susan Bell

KYLE BOOKS

An Hachette UK Company
www.hachette.co.uk

First published in Great Britain in 2019 by
Kyle Books, an imprint of Kyle Cathie Ltd
Carmelite House
50 Victoria Embankment
London EC4Y 0DZ
www.kylebooks.co.uk

ISBN: 978 0 85783 622 9/978 0 85783 449 2

Distributed in the US by Hachette Book Group, 1290 Avenue of the Americas,
4th and 5th Floors, New York, NY 10104

Distributed in Canada by Canadian Manda Group, 664 Annette St., Toronto, Ontario, Canada M6S 2C8

Editor: Vicky Orchard
Design: Tina Smith Hobson
Photography: Susan Bell
Food and props styling: Susie Theodorou
Production: Emily Noto

A Cataloguing in Publication record for this title is available from the British Library

Printed and bound in Italy

10 9

NOTE: The information in this book is only part of how any particular person may decide which diet or indeed lifestyle is the best for them. If you are on prescribed medication or suffer from a significant medical condition we strongly advise you to consult your own doctor before making changes. For example improvements in lifestyle and weight loss may also significantly improve your blood pressure or diabetes control requiring a reduction in medication.
The science part of this book is written from the viewpoint of people with type 2 diabetes or those wishing to lose weight. The recipes may also be suitable for people with type 1 diabetes provided of course that you consult your doctor as advised above.

CONTENTS

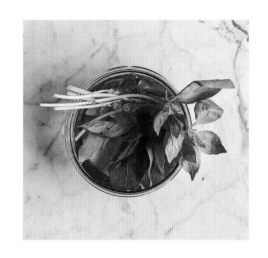

Introduction

Recipes

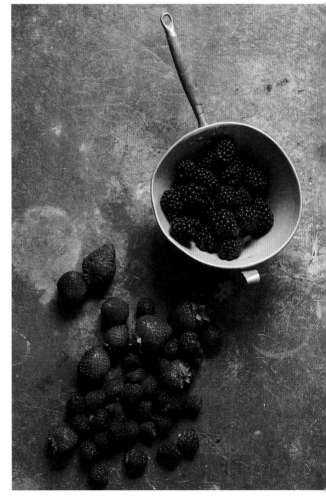

Foreword by Dr David Unwin FRCGP

"I believe we have eaten our way into this epidemic of diabetes and obesity and that we can eat our way out of it."

I decided to help with the development of this book for two reasons. Firstly, I see it as part of a very exciting worldwide revolution; where a low-carb approach to diet is helping people with type 2 diabetes and obesity to take control of their health. Secondly, I recognize that Katie and Giancarlo know all about producing great food, but, far more importantly, that Giancarlo's own diabetes story is so similar to that of many of my patients that I feel they have the necessary health insights to produce a really useful book.

My Eureka Moment

Just after I joined my Southport GP practice in 1986, we did a survey of our patients with type 2 diabetes; there were just 57 cases. At the time, we called this either "sugar diabetes" or "maturity onset diabetes" to reflect the fact that it usually developed in people in their mid-sixties or later, and that sugar was agreed to be part of its causation. Our practice had no patients with type 2 diabetes under the age of 50.

Now, 40 years on, we have gone from 57 patients with type 2 diabetes to 472! Twenty-one of these patients are under 50, with an average body weight of 110kg (17.5 stone). The youngest is 34. So I have seen more than a eight-fold increase in the prevalence of diagnosed diabetes, and the patients are getting steadily younger.

For the first 25 years, I didn't think there was much that could be done about this depressing trend. It seemed to be largely a matter of adding in more drugs or increasing dosages. Then one day about six years ago everything changed. I met a lady who had lost so much weight that I didn't recognize her, and when we did blood tests she had reversed her type 2 diabetes (remission might be a better word); and this despite coming off her diabetes medication! I was fascinated, having not seen a single case of diabetes remission in my medical career. How had she achieved this? The lady explained she was one of 40,000 members of a low-carb forum on the Diabetes.co.uk website. This began my own journey of discovery.

My wife Jen and I started a low-carb group in my GP practice and, together with our practice nurse Heather, we trialled a low-carb diet. Along with 18 volunteer patients, we met each Monday night and learned about low-carb together. The results were eventually published and, since then, the offer of a lower carb approach to type 2 diabetes has been taken up by hundreds of patients in our practice. This has resulted in us prescribing far less

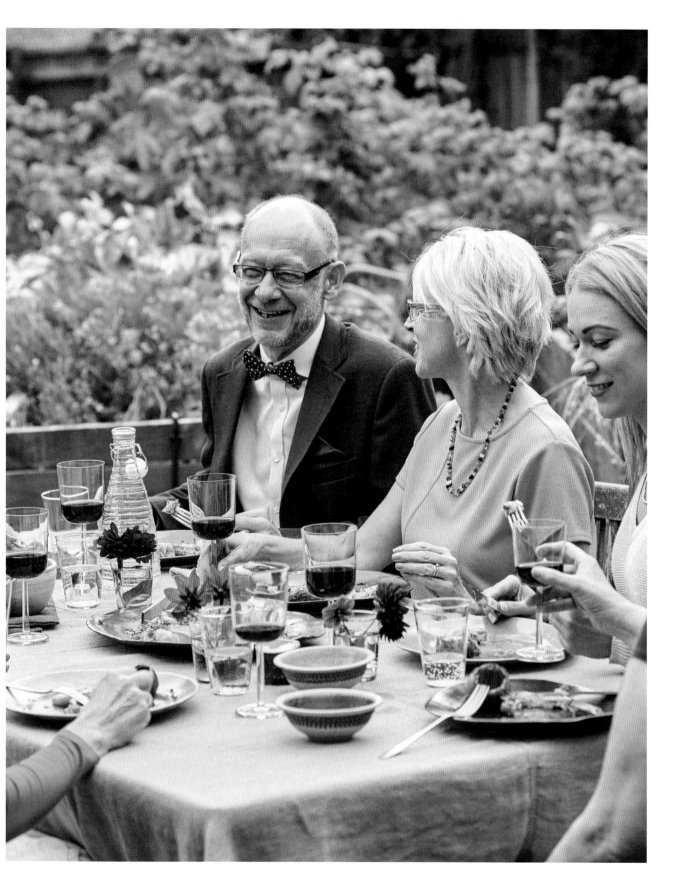

medication for diabetes than is average in our area – about £40,000 per year. It was for this work in 2016 that I was named NHS Innovator of the Year, and then in 2018 we were shortlisted for GP Practice of the Year.

Now I don't accept this epidemic of diabetes is inevitable or hopeless. My patients' genes haven't changed in 30 years; only the environment acting upon a genetic predisposition. Although stress and lack of exercise are co-factors, I have come to feel that the most important cause of "sugar diabetes" is diet. Surely this is a hopeful message because we all have some control over our dietary choices, producing a great opportunity to turn back the clock on obesity and diabetes.

Essentially people with type 2 diabetes have a problem dealing with sugar, or glucose. This is why it builds up in the bloodstream, resulting in higher than normal blood sugars which, over time, damage small blood vessels in vital organs. From this it would

seem obvious to cut sugar out of the diet – if possible completely – particularly as we don't actually need any dietary sugar at all. In many cases, this simple first step can make a huge difference and may render the use of lifelong drugs for diabetes unnecessary. I have seen the total elimination of sugar improve not just diabetes but also blood pressure, liver function and even mood in many cases. I have heard it said that sugar may be okay 'in moderation'. This worries me for two reasons: firstly, if we don't need to eat any sugar, eating even a moderate amount could leave someone with type 2 diabetes "moderately poisoned" quite unnecessarily. Secondly, I find in practice sugar addiction is a serious problem. If you are a sugar addict it may be very difficult to have just one biscuit, or you may find a single square of milk chocolate generates powerful cravings for more!

Often I come across patients who wonder why they still have diabetes when they have already cut out sugar completely. However, most people only think of

How starchy carbs affect blood sugar levels

Food item	G Index	Serve size (g)	How does each food affect blood glucose compared with one 4g teaspoon of table sugar?
Basmati rice	69	150	10.1
Potato, white, boiled	96	150	9.1
French fries, baked	64	150	7.5
Spaghetti, white, boiled	39	180	6.6
Sweetcorn, boiled	60	80	4.0
Frozen peas, boiled	51	80	1.3
Banana	62	120	5.7
Apple	39	120	2.3
Slice of wholemeal bread	74	30	3.0
Broccoli	15	80	0.2
Eggs	0	60	0

From Unwin et al (2016). It is the glycaemic response to, not the carbohydrate content of food that matters in diabetes. The glycaemic index revisited. Journal of Insulin Resistance.

> **"you can see that a banana is likely to produce nearly three times more sugar than an apple"**

the obvious sources of sugar, like sweetened drinks or chocolate bars, missing the important fact that starchy carbohydrates such as bread, rice or potatoes digest down into surprising amounts of glucose. For example, one 30g (1oz) slice of brown bread affects blood glucose to the same extent as 3 teaspoons of sugar, or a 150g (5oz) baked potato as much as 8 teaspoons of sugar. This explains why the latest English type 2 diabetes guidelines state:

● Encourage high fibre, low glycaemic index sources of carbohydrate in the diet.
● Individualize recommendations for carbohydrate and alcohol intake.

The challenges are how to implement these guidelines in practice, and how best to explain what 'low-glycaemic-index carbohydrates' means.

The glycaemic index (GI) ranks the carbohydrates in our foods to give us an idea of just how much sugar starchy carbs produce as they are digested down, compared to a meal of pure glucose. Nearly all breads and cereals have a high GI compared to green veg, most nuts or eggs. Many people with type 2 diabetes find it helps to "turn the white part of your meal green". So, instead of steak and chips, try steak and loads of coleslaw, salad or broccoli. Another example is to replace the rice with your curry with green beans, asparagus or cauliflower, pouring the curry sauce over a big pile of veg instead of rice.

A few years ago, with a well-known academic in the field, Dr Geoffrey Livesey, I produced a new system of "teaspoon of table sugar equivalents" in an attempt

to help people understand what may happen to their blood sugar after eating various carbohydrate foods and then make better dietary choices. The idea is to compare a serving of a particular food to its equivalent in terms of teaspoons of sugar (see table opposite).

Looking at the table opposite you can see that a banana is likely to produce about three times more sugar than an apple and that it might be better for someone with type 2 diabetes to have more green veg instead of potatoes, bread or rice.

Five years ago, I started encouraging my patients that it wasn't hopeless, that they could make real health improvements if they were prepared to look seriously at reducing all dietary sources of glucose. Many of them were particularly interested in a losing weight or avoiding lifelong medication. Some of my patients have kindly consented to me sharing their data, so I now have 86 very proud patients who, at the time of writing, have been on a low-carb diet for an average of 20 months, with significant average improvements in diabetes and blood pressure control, weight (an average of about 9kg (nearly 20lb) weight loss), cholesterol and lipid profiles.

The table opposite gives an idea of how I have used the teaspoon equivalent system to help my patients understand why a low-carb breakfast of scrambled eggs or full-fat yogurt and blueberries may be a better choice for them than the traditional toast or high-sugar breakfast cereals.

It would not be fair to say this is all my idea. Cutting carbs or a "low-carb diet" has a worldwide following, and not just among diabetics. Of course, no one diet will suit everyone, and for the sake of balance, I should point out that there are experts who worry about low-carb diets in the long-term, though over the five years I have been using a low-carb diet with my patients, I haven't come across any significant problems. An Austrian consultant specialist Dr Wolfgang Lutz was on the diet for 40 years until his death aged 96 and used the approach to help his patients for decades. This was the basis for his fascinating book, *Life Without Bread: How a Low-Carbohydrate Diet Can Save Your Life.*

It's not just about diabetes; belly fat matters

Our bodies respond to a sugary meal by producing the hormone insulin, which pushes the sugar into muscle cells for energy. Excess sugar is pushed into belly fat and the liver. Over time, as we take in more sugar than we need, central obesity and fatty liver disease result. At least 20 per cent of the developed world now has fatty liver disease. I worry that excess sugar and starchy carbs are leading to the three great modern epidemics: diabetes, obesity and fatty liver disease. In 2000, the World Health Organization concluded there was convincing evidence that central obesity (defined as a waist greater than 80cm/31.5in) in women or 94cm/37in) in men) was associated with significantly increased risk of:
- Cardiovascular disease
- Hypertension
- Colorectal and breast cancer
- Overall mortality

The good news is that I have often seen a low-carb

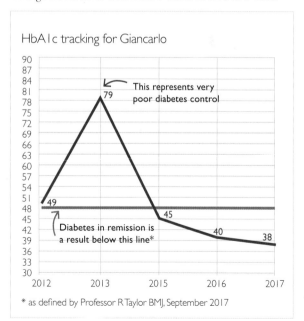

HbA1c tracking for Giancarlo

79 — This represents very poor diabetes control

49

45

40

38

Diabetes in remission is a result below this line*

2012   2013   2015   2016   2017

* as defined by Professor R Taylor BMJ, September 2017

approach help not just type 2 diabetes but also liver function, blood pressure, lipid profiles (particularly triglyceride and HDL cholesterol levels) and central obesity. One of my patients even coined the phrase "low-carb liposuction" he was so pleased with his improved appearance!

Giancarlo's Story

In my first 25 years as a GP, I had never seen diabetes go into remission, but I am delighted to say that it's something I see most weeks now in my clinical practice as people with type 2 diabetes and obesity learn how to avoid dietary sugar and starchy carbs. Giancarlo's story is particularly impressive, as the graph of his HbA1c (see left) shows. The HbA1c is a blood test we do to give an idea of average blood sugar control over the preceding few months. A higher result would indicate poor control, as shown by Giancarlo's result of 79 mmol/mol in 2013. Anything under 48 is no longer in the diabetic range.

By 2013 Giancarlo's diabetic control was really bad and he weighed 108kg (17st), but by 2017 he had lost 19kg (3st) and had a normal blood sugar; his diabetes was in medication-free remission! Before changing his diet he also had oddly numb feet, because of a complication of more severe diabetes called "peripheral neuropathy", where the persistently raised blood sugars affect the long nerves – usually those going to the feet – resulting in numbness. Giancarlo is unusual in that his is just the third case where I have seen this particular diabetic complication resolve, each time with a low-carb diet.

In the last five years I have seen a low carbohydrate diet help many patients come off medication and take control of their health. I do hope I have explained why I find this diet so interesting, and why quite apart from the delicious recipes this book may be of interest to you too!

Follow me on Twitter @lowcarbGP

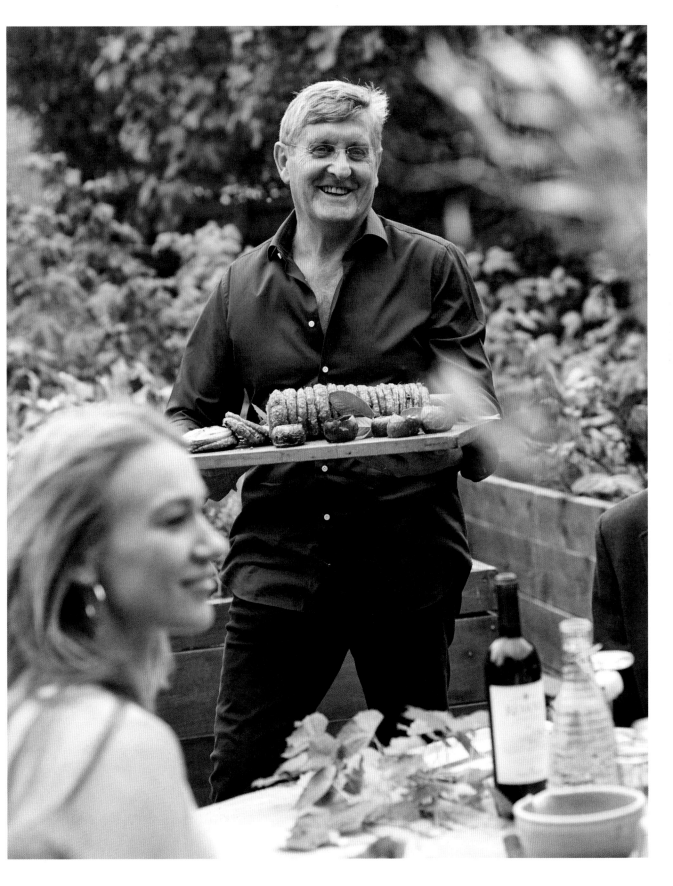

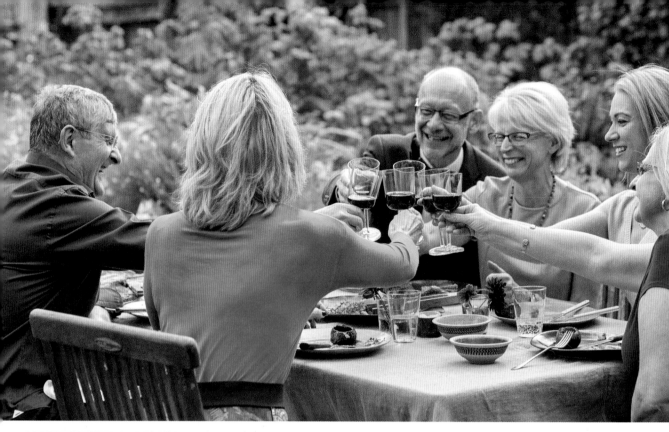

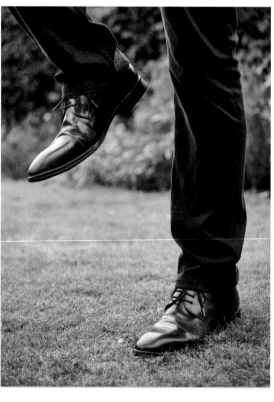

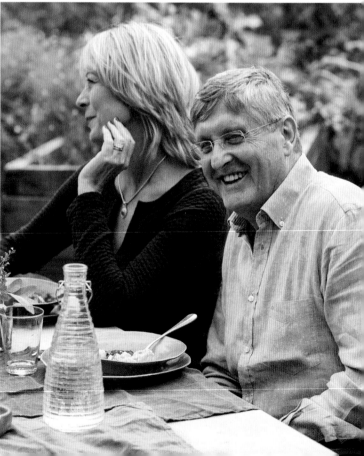

Introduction: OUR STORIES

Giancarlo's Journey to Diabetes Remission

Ten years after the millennium celebrations, Giancarlo and I should have been in a good place. We had two children, two restaurants, a cookery school and a series of cookbooks to our name. A BBC2 television series called *Return to Tuscany* had been made about our lives, and Giancarlo had been awarded the honour of Cavaliere del Lavoro by the Italian government for his work in promoting Italian food.

However, we hadn't realized that a grey and menacing cloud was slowly moving over our world. Looking back, it took years to take effect and appeared so quietly we simply didn't see it. The successful, energetic, larger-than-life character that I had fallen in love with 15 years before had been replaced with an overweight, moody, tired and listless shell of his former self. When I met Giancarlo, he was known as Tigger from *Winnie the Pooh* by the customers at the restaurant, but over the years he had become a lot more like Eeyore, the sad and slow donkey from the same story. He weighed just over 100kg (16st), had frequent and excruciating attacks of gout, constant arthritis in his hands and knees, was always thirsty, had to nap several times a day and everything was an effort. He would become hungry and angry and then gorge on fruit, sugary cappuccinos or huge, oversized bowls of spaghetti, often being so "hangry" he would eat straight from the saucepan. Then came disturbing bouts of blurred vision and blackouts. It was only then he took himself to the doctor. After routine blood tests, he was called back for the results.

In 2011, Giancarlo was told he had type 2 diabetes.

Not understanding the seriousness of the condition, we probably didn't react quickly enough. Giancarlo followed his dietician's advice to eat smaller portions of food and cut back on sugar. The dietician also measured my waist size and warned me that as I was overweight I was in danger of being pre-diabetic. We didn't eat processed foods and cooked everything from scratch, so we couldn't see where we were going wrong. Over the following three years neither of us lost weight and Giancarlo's blood sugar levels rose. He looked and felt even worse.

By 2013, Giancarlo weighed 108kg (17st) and was suffering with numb feet that made playing football with the kids or climbing stairs difficult. His HbA1c level (average blood sugar count) was 79mmol/mol (non-diabetic is less than 48). In 2014, there was a lot in the press about gluten intolerance, and I wondered whether if we cut out white flour from our diet, the lack of gluten would help us lose weight and stop my bloated tummy. It didn't make any difference to me, but after three days, Giancarlo felt amazing. We went to see Jenny Phillips, a superb nutritionist, and after blood tests she confirmed he had a severe gluten intolerance. When Jenny told him, it felt like his world of food and everything he loved was forbidden. Although determined to fight, he felt very low. No pasta, no pizza, no choux buns or bread. Imagine an Italian man who, over almost 60 years, was used to eating his beloved pasta at least once, and often twice, a day being told to stop. What Giancarlo didn't realize at the time is that this diagnosis would probably save his life.

As soon as Giancarlo gave up wheat, and therefore dramatically reduced the carbohydrate part of

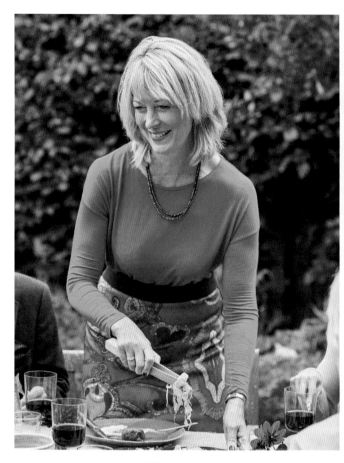

his meals, he felt better: the swelling in his joints disappeared, his blood sugar levels dropped and he began to lose weight. He stopped eating pasta, found alternatives to pastry, bread and pizza, and made a point not to load up with rice or potatoes instead.

At this time, we started to write our book *Around the World in Salads*, which meant we were constantly testing recipes made up primarily of salad leaves, herbs and vegetables. To this we would add meat, fish or dairy protein, and fat in the way of salad dressings.

Inadvertently, we were following a low-carb diet. I was constantly online searching for information and recipes and came across a world of low-carb eaters and, most importantly, low-carb eaters who had type 2 diabetes and who had turned their condition around. Through the site Diabetes.co.uk we became familiar with the name of Dr David Unwin who, with his wife Dr Jen Unwin, held a clinic to support people with type 2 diabetes and other conditions that can be helped by a low-carb diet. Giancarlo, Jenny and I were keen to learn more about their work and we soon met up to swap stories. This book is the result of that encounter – our common goal was to provide a clear explanation of the facts, backed up by medical and nutritional knowledge, as well as easy-to-follow recipes to demonstrate the wonderful food we all love to eat. We have a joint love of food; we are greedy and love mealtimes. Giancarlo and I are surrounded by food and, if we can manage to stay slim and healthy, so can you!

Now, seven years on from Giancarlo's first diabetes diagnosis, he has lost 19kg (3st) and his HbA1c levels have dropped to normal, just 38mmol/mol. His diabetes is in full remission! He has gone from a man who couldn't tie his own shoelaces (he couldn't reach his feet) to a man who can once again enjoy an active life with his family and dog. He even runs upstairs now the odd numbness in his feet has gone! I have shed over a stone in weight and have kept it off. It's been a difficult journey, but it's never too late to make a start. (See more about Giancarlo's story at www.caldesi.com.)

"I could see patterns in Giancarlo's eating and still can. Now I, too, have my glucose levels under control I can be so much stronger and don't crave food all the time. Low-carb suits us both."

My Conversion to Low-Carb

(Jenny Phillips mBANT
www.InspiredNutrition.co.uk)

My route into low-carb eating wasn't due to diabetes. My health crisis came at the age of just 39 when, as a mum of two young children, I had the devastating diagnosis of breast cancer.

Up until that point, I would have told you that I was healthy and had a good diet. In reality, I was taking a number of medications, thinking at the time that this was completely normal. I rigidly followed healthy eating guidelines such as high starch, low fat and low salt.

My diagnosis changed everything. I was fortunate in that the medical treatment was successful, but I wanted to learn more about how I could prevent a recurrence. With a first degree in chemistry, I was at an advantage to explore the science surrounding health and nutrition, and became engrossed in the fascinating world of human health. I went on to qualify with a further degree in Nutritional Medicine and also trained as a yoga teacher.

My studies opened up a new world and I was quick to make changes to my diet. Out went the 'not-so-healthy' eating guidelines and I was instead guided by a focus on real foods and ingredients. It became very apparent to me that sugar and processed and refined carbs were not helping and, as these came out of my diet, my health soared to new levels. In a short space of time I no longer needed meds to manage asthma, hay fever and indigestion. Headaches and period pains resolved as if by magic. I lost weight naturally, my sleep improved and my energy levels increased dramatically.

The other reason that my new low-carb diet was so compelling is that I learned that sugar feeds cancer cells. There is much more detail in my book, *Eat to Outsmart Cancer*, but suffice to say that cancer cells make energy by the fermentation of sugar. This process is called "glycolysis" and should be made known to all concerned when recovering from, or preventing, cancer.

For the last 10 years, I have been working with clients like Giancarlo and Katie, and have the privilege of helping people to improve their own health through nutrition, exercise and lifestyle.

> "In a short space of time
> I no longer needed meds
> to manage asthma, hay fever
> and indigestion."

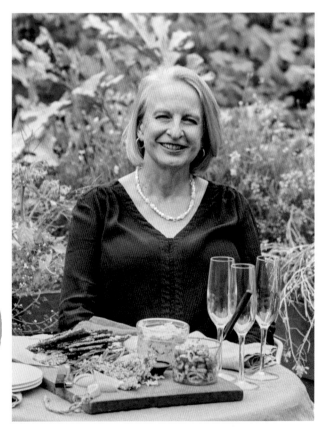

Unlocking THE REAL SCIENCE

By Jenny Phillips, Nutritional Therapist

When did eating become so complicated?

There is a growing awareness that food is directly related to our health. Indeed, it is now frequently described as medicine. However, there seems to be a wide variety of opinions on the subject, which are often conflicting. This can leave you feeling unsure of what to do for the best, which can mean continuing with an eating pattern even if it doesn't help with your health goals or the way that you feel.

You may be aware of the current healthy eating advice, which encourages you to "base meals on starchy carbohydrates" such as bread, pasta, potatoes, rice and cereals. The trouble is that these starchy foods break down into glucose, potentially causing blood sugar problems and weight gain.

The recommended carbohydrate intake is at least 250g (9oz), which we feel is incredibly high for most people. If you are aiming to manage your blood sugars better, or to lose weight, then this may be up to five times more carbs than your body can handle.

As a nutritionist I see numerous food diaries, and most people are following this advice. I did too before my "health revolution" in 2003: cereals for breakfast, sandwiches for lunch, and a dinner with potatoes, rice or pasta.

There is now a growing body of medical practitioners, such as Dr Unwin, who are recommending dietary advice which is more effective at managing type 2 diabetes (importantly this is recognized within the NHS, although not all doctors are aware of it). This involves restricting starchy carbohydrates, the very foods that cause an increase in blood glucose. Most nutritionists (and many dieticians) agree wholeheartedly, and confirm that this approach is also beneficial for weight loss.

How Much Sugar?

An effective way to familiarize yourself with how certain foods affect your blood sugar levels is to take a look at the "sugar equivalent" infographics that Dr Unwin has discussed in his foreword. These are a powerful way to see just how sugary many popular starchy foods are. You may well be familiar with "sugar equivalents" in respect of foods with a high sugar content, such as a can of cola containing nine teaspoons of sugar. But you might find this information both surprising and shocking when applied to popular foods that you could well be consuming regularly. The chart opposite can help to produce a 'light bulb' moment, which may explain why your current diet is not helping you to lose weight or improve blood sugars.

We've also added the carbohydrate content, as this will help you in respect of tracking your carb intake. In addition to the carb content, the sugar equivalents utilize the glycaemic index (GI), which predicts how much a food affects blood glucose levels.

How starchy carbs affect your blood sugar levels

Cereal (serving size 30g)	Carb g	G Index	How does each cereal affect blood glucose compared to 4g teaspoon of table sugar?
Coco Pops	26	77	7.3
Corn Flakes	25	93	8.4
Mini wheats	20	59	4.4
Shredded Wheat	20	67	4.8
Special K	20	54	4
Bran Flakes	18	74	4.8
Oat porridge	19	63	4.4
Bread (serving size 30g)			
White bread	14	71	3.7
Brown bread	12	74	3.3
Rye (69% wholegrain rye flour)	14	78	4
Wholegrain barley (50% barley)	18	85	5.5
Wholemeal stoneground	12	59	2.6
Pitta wholemeal	14	56	2.9
Oatmeal batch	15	62	3.3
Fruit (serving size 120g)			
Banana	26	62	5.9
Grapes, black	19	59	4
Apple (Golden Delicious)	15	39	2.2
Watermelon	6	80	1.8
Nectarines	10	43	1.5
Apricots	9	34	1.1
Strawberries	6	40	0.4
Common foods			
Basmati rice 150g	40	69	10.1
Potato, white 150g	26	96	9.1
French fries 150g	32	64	7.5
Spaghetti, white 180g	46	39	6.6
Sweetcorn 80g	18	60	4
Frozen peas 80g	7	51	1.3
Broccoli 80g	4	15	0.2
Eggs 60g	0	0	0

Sugar is Everywhere

Carbohydrates, or carbs, are one of three food macronutrients, along with fats and protein. There are two main types – sugars (which tend to have names ending in -ose like glucose, lactose and fructose) and starches (found in grains including wheat, rice, potato, cereals and vegetables).

Now just about everyone knows that consuming sugar – in cakes, biscuits, sweets and milk chocolate – is bad news for managing type 2 diabetes and losing weight. These foods cause a surge in blood sugar levels and often lead to weight gain. But did you know that starchy foods are made up of strings of sugar molecules, which are broken down by digestion and absorbed into the bloodstream in exactly the same way? This is why these foods can have exactly the same effect as eating sugar and are a particular issue for someone who is trying to lose weight or who is diabetic. The starchier the food, the more sugar molecules it contains and the faster it raises blood sugar levels.

Many of the savoury foods that are eaten regularly (like sandwiches, pasta, pizza, crisps and pies) are extremely starchy. They release a lot of sugar molecules very quickly.

Vegetables can be divided into two camps:

1. Starchy veg: vegetables that have a higher starch content, including many of the vegetables that grow below ground, such as potatoes, sweet potatoes, carrots and parsnips.
2. Non-starchy veg: the vast range of mostly above-ground vegetables like leafy greens and salad vegetables.

Non-starchy veg can be eaten generously without adversely affecting blood glucose levels. For a full list of which vegetables can be eaten only in moderation (starchy) or generously (non-starchy) see the food plan on page 39. The image on pages 37–38 shows the scale of vegetables from low carb to high carb.

Many processed foods contain lots of sugar in addition to starches (which break down into sugar). One study estimates that up to a whopping 74 per

> "If only type 2 diabetes was known as 'carbohydrate intolerance'."

cent of packaged foods and beverages include added sugar or sweeteners to enhance their taste.

Even foods that are promoted with low-fat messages or healthy looking packaging can be high in total carbs and sugars. The table below shows some common supermarket foods which have a higher carbohydrate content per serving than a chocolate bar. As you can see, it's important to always read the label!

Type 2 diabetes is effectively a condition of carbohydrate intolerance. When sugary or starchy foods are eaten, the body is not able to manage the flood of sugar into the blood and hence blood glucose levels rise. The solution? Follow the guidelines in this book to learn about managing your carbohydrate intake according to your own tolerance.

It's not just people who have been diagnosed with diabetes that need to worry about their carbohydrate intake – blood sugar spikes are not good for anyone, especially if you want to keep your energy levels, mood and weight stable.

Popular foods can be high in carbs				
	Serving size	kcal	Carbs (g)	Sugar (g)
'Healthy' cereal	30g	114	25.4	4.6
Low-fat vanilla yogurt	150g	135	20.7	20.4
Low-fat custard	130g	116	20	14.3
Energy bar	35g	135	18.2	16.6
Milk chocolate	32.5g	174	18	18

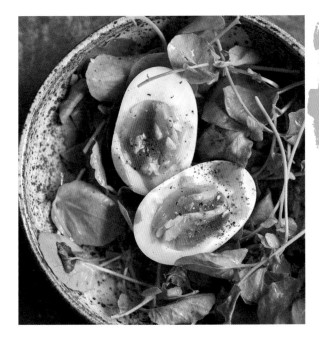

Yes, you heard that right; insulin is also a fat storage hormone. This helps to explain why weight gain, especially around the middle, is common in type 2 diabetics, affecting 9 out of 10 sufferers.

When you regularly eat high-starch foods, which may include many foods that you believe to be good for you, such as cereal or wholemeal toast, your blood sugar and insulin spike too high and too often. You gain weight, but you also feel the effects of a "sugar dip" as insulin overreacts to bring sugar levels crashing down. You may recognize this as tiredness and lethargy.

The Blood Sugar Rollercoaster

You might be surprised at how little glucose is in your bloodstream normally – typically up to 2 teaspoons. Just imagine, then, that you eat something really starchy, like a doughnut or a bowl of rice. Once in your digestive system, powerful enzymes get to work to break the starch down into glucose molecules. These are absorbed into your bloodstream. High-starch foods release a lot of sugar very quickly, and this drives your blood sugar upwards. You can measure this using a blood glucose monitor, such as a FreeStyle Libre device, where you will see this as a spike in your blood sugar.

In response to this sugar surge, your pancreas releases insulin. This hormone is the master controller of glucose, moving it into the body's cells to be used as fuel for energy. Any that is surplus to requirements is moved to the liver and converted into glycogen as an energy reserve, or stored as fat.

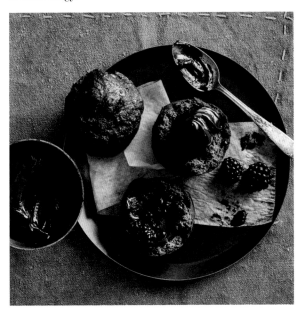

In this weakened position, feeling tired and fed up, you often reach for another "pick-me-up", such as a chocolate bar or a couple of biscuits. This vicious cycle leads to overeating, as high-starch foods push up your blood sugar which provokes an insulin rush. The excess sugar is converted into fat, leading to an energy crash and strong cravings for sweet and starchy foods. You berate yourself for being weak-willed, but you are an animal being driven by hormones.

In the long term, blood sugar control issues are likely to arise, which is why we currently have an epidemic of diabesity (type 2 diabetes and obesity). Constant grazing and an obsession with sweet and starchy foods can lead to "insulin resistance", where the cells don't respond as they should. Your body reacts by producing more and more insulin to force sugar out of the bloodstream. Once the cells are truly overloaded, despite having high insulin levels, glucose will remain there – it has nowhere else to go. Your body can no longer handle carbohydrates well and, once blood glucose levels cannot be maintained in the normal range, you are diagnosed as type 2 diabetic.

We really need to get into a virtuous cycle, adopting a diet of low-carbohydrate foods combined with healthy protein and fat. As an example, eating a handful of nuts as a snack rather than a biscuit or two will have a minimal impact on your blood sugar levels, preventing a blood sugar and then insulin spike, and will sustain you for longer. We want to encourage you to choose real foods which are rich in colour and variety, without the predominance of refined and heavily processed foods that are now synonymous with causing so many health issues.

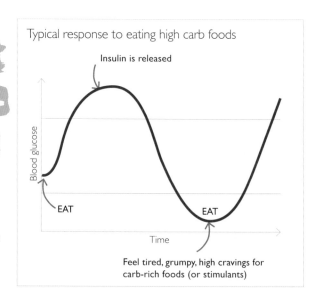

Typical response to eating high carb foods

Insulin is released

Blood glucose

EAT

EAT

Time

Feel tired, grumpy, high cravings for carb-rich foods (or stimulants)

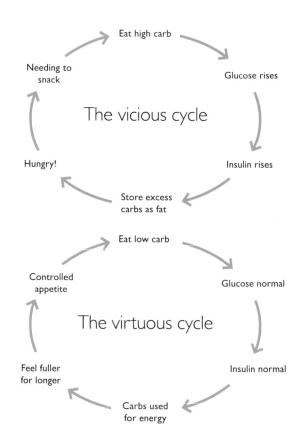

Eat high carb

Glucose rises

Needing to snack

The vicious cycle

Insulin rises

Hungry!

Store excess carbs as fat

Eat low carb

Controlled appetite

Glucose normal

The virtuous cycle

Insulin normal

Feel fuller for longer

Carbs used for energy

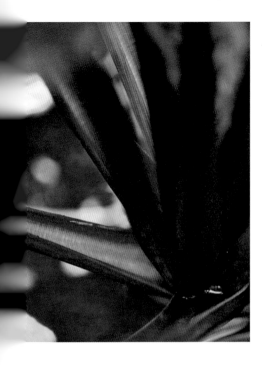

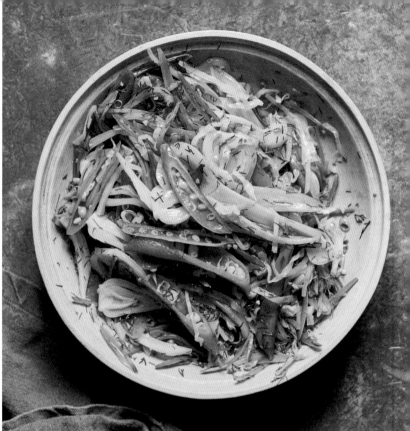

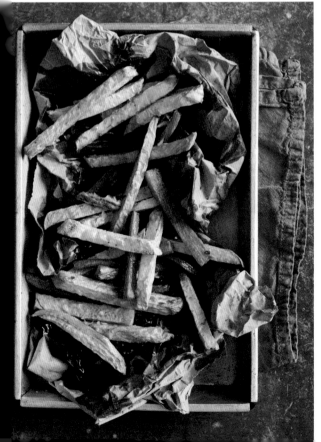

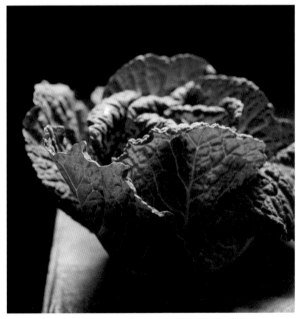

Low Carb vs Low Calorie

It is now clear why low-carb improves blood sugar levels: restricting sugar and starchy carbohydrate reduces spikes in blood glucose and allows insulin levels to normalize. Without the insulin rush, you feel more satisfied after meals and this helps to moderate your appetite. Lower insulin levels allow you to burn body fat, which can be enhanced when combined with intermittent fasting (see page 26). This is crucial if you want to lose weight, and also means that you feel good because you are not suffering from swings in your energy supply. Fat is your alternative fuel.

For many people, a low-carb diet is far more effective than eating low-calorie foods, which are typically low in fat but high in insulin-spiking refined carbs and added sugars. These foods also tend to be highly processed and do not sustain or nourish you. A good example is a snack pack containing two chocolate covered rice cakes which many of you may consider a healthy choice: the packaging boldly states "only 81 calories". A closer inspection of the nutrition label reveals that these contain 67g of carbs per 100g. This is way too carby if your aim is to manage blood sugar levels well.

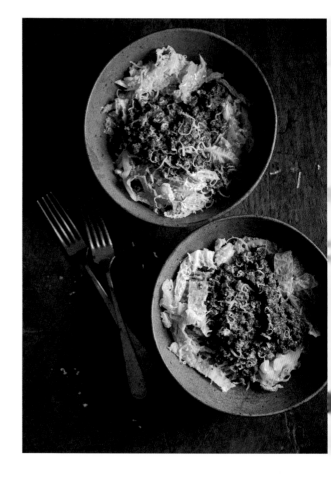

Fat as an alternative fuel

Fat   Carbs

Glucose

Acetyl CoA

Energy

LOW-CARB NOT NO-CARB
Low-carb is the colloquial term for describing a diet that restricts both sugars and starchy carbohydrates.

The aim of this book is to demonstrate why low-carb is a very helpful food philosophy for good health. However, we don't believe there is a "one-size-fits-all" recommendation to how low you should go. It all depends on your overall health and what your goals are; we encourage you to experiment with the level that best suits you. So we have developed the CarbScale (see opposite) – a way of flexing your carb intake rather than shunning this entire food group.

As you would expect from a cookbook, our focus is on fresh foods and ingredients. We recognize that this may require you to spend more time preparing food than you do at the moment, which is why we've made it easy in the recipes that follow. Before we get started though, let's delve a little deeper into the approach and guide you through how this book can best be used to regain control of your own health.

YOUR NEW
CarbScale MENU

The CarbScale is our plan which restricts high GI (glycaemic index) foods, such as grains, cereals, starchy vegetables and some fruits, which digest down into rather surprising amounts of sugar and, of course, sugar itself. Instead, it puts the emphasis on ingredients rich in protein and healthy fats, as well as low-glycaemic fruit and abundant green, leafy and salad vegetables. We refer to a scale because this allows you to flex the plan to meet your individual needs, rather than following a 'one-size-fits-all' formula. It refers to the target amount of carbohydrates you will eat in a day. Take our quick quiz to learn more about your metabolism, which is the process of how you make energy from food, and where you currently are on the CarbScale.

Where are you on the CarbScale?

Just rate each of the following statements from 1 = strongly disagree to 5 = strongly agree

I feel tired a lot of the time	1	2	3	4	5
I often wake up feeling tired	1	2	3	4	5
My energy slumps in the day	1	2	3	4	5
I constantly crave sweet or savoury foods	1	2	3	4	5
I rely on coffee to perk me up	1	2	3	4	5
I like something sweet after a meal	1	2	3	4	5
I want to lose weight	1	2	3	4	5
My mood is low or depressed	1	2	3	4	5
I often feel anxious or stressed	1	2	3	4	5
I'm finding it hard to lose weight	1	2	3	4	5
I don't sleep well	1	2	3	4	5
I can get irritable between meals	1	2	3	4	5

Your score

NOW ADD UP YOUR SCORES:
below 18 = Liberal low carb
Congratulations – you are doing a great job! Your metabolism is generally working well and you are feeling pretty good. Low carb is still right for you because it is a fantastic way to achieve a varied and nutritious diet, but you can afford a little more flexibility, particularly if you have high levels of exercise.

19–47 = Moderate low carb
Generally life is treating you well, but you still have some health goals to accomplish. Your metabolism may benefit from some fine tuning so that you feel more energized and focused. As you start to include some of the low carb and nutritious recipes and ideas in this book, monitor how you feel to keep yourself on track.

48+ = Strict low carb
You may have health issues that you are trying to work through. It is likely that your metabolism has slowed down and you may be finding it hard to achieve all you need to in the day. Chances are that you have a degree of carbohydrate intolerance, and foods like breads, rice, and pasta will cause rapid swings in your blood sugars. Try to focus on excluding high carbohydrate foods, whilst enjoying new recipes from this book.

The Seven CarbScale principles

Below is a summary of the principles of the CarbScale based on a slightly stricter carbohydrate target (like the one Giancarlo follows), which we encourage you to experiment with.

If you are lean and healthy, then these principles are still valid, but you can afford slightly more leeway. Jenny tends to add in extra fruit and starchy vegetables, whereas Katie prefers the occasional slice of sourdough bread or a small bowl of pasta.

1 **Reduce or eliminate sugar and starchy carbohydrate foods.** These include: breakfast cereals, bread, pasta, white potatoes, rice, couscous, crackers, oats, oat cakes, rice cakes, cakes, biscuits, sweets, milk chocolate, fruit juice, fizzy drinks and cordials.

2 **Load up with vegetables at each meal.** Non-starchy and salad vegetables should be eaten generously so that you feel full at each meal. Eat root vegetables depending on your carbohydrate tolerance (where you are on the CarbScale).

3 **Include good fats within your diet** – these are essential for your metabolism and help you to feel fuller for longer. Include oily fish, olive oil, coconut oil, avocado and animal fats. Nuts and cheese can be added in moderation; they are nutritious and tasty but also highly calorific, so go easy on them.

4 **When it comes to fruit, berries are good** as they are naturally low in sugar. Take a look at the photo on pages 36–37 which shows the range of fruits from low to high carb. Try to avoid high-sugar tropical fruits, such as mango, pineapple and banana.

5 **Enjoy protein with every meal** – it's essential to your body and helps you feel fuller for longer.

6 **Stop snacking.** Fasting between meals and overnight can really help to improve insulin resistance – we are not designed to eat constantly! Aim for three good meals a day and then stop.

7 **Drink about 2 litres (3½ pints) of water a day.**

How Low (in Carbs) Should You Go?

Within the low-carb community there are broadly three tiers of intake which suit different people. Depending on your own metabolism, once you have an idea of where you sit on the CarbScale, you can experiment with the following:

1. Liberal low-carb: up to 130g (4½oz) carbs per day. Suitable for those who are lean and healthy, with an active lifestyle.
2. Moderate low-carb: 75–100g (2¾–3½oz) carbs per day. This enables a wide and varied diet and is a good starting point into carbohydrate restriction. It is also a good target for the long-term as it is not too restrictive.
3. Strict low-carb: limiting dietary carbohydrate to about 50g (2oz) per day affords even tighter glycaemic control and is a reasonable therapeutic aim for type 2 diabetics and those suffering with low energy or cravings.

If you have high activity levels and are lean, fit and healthy, then you may wish to retain some higher starch foods within your diet. However, to achieve health benefits, your overall diet should contain sufficient high-quality food, including protein, healthy fat and mostly unprocessed, slow-release carbohydrates, such as oats and starchy vegetables, like sweet potatoes, beetroot and pulses. Even for athletes, the days of heavy carb-loading are waning – England Rugby, for example, encourages its players to consume lots of vegetables and protein in addition to slow-release carbohydrates.

DO I REALLY NEED TO WEIGH MY FOOD?
No. You may just decide to swap out some of your high carb foods, like bread, rice and pasta, for extra vegetables and see how this works for you. However, at the start it can be really helpful to have a rough idea of your daily carb count so that you can make adjustments as you go along. Don't panic though as there are several ways to estimate your carb intake.

Individualising the plan – the Caldesi team

	Giancarlo	Katie	Jenny	Natalia
Health goal	Reversed diabetes. Must keep weight off for health reasons.	Watching waist measurement stays below 80cm (31.5in)	Weight maintenance and energy. Lots of exercise.	Maintain athletic performance; balance hormones.
Daily carb intake	About 50g (2oz)	Under 75g (2¾oz)	Under 100g (3½oz)	About 130g (4½oz)
Meat	Lots	Lots	Moderate	Occasionally
Fish	Lots	Lots	Twice a week	Most days
Dairy	Occasionally	Most days	Most days	Most days
Eggs	Every day	Every day	Often	Every day
Grains	Never	Once a week	Occasional oats or buckwheat only	Most days – porridge or sourdough bread
Pulses	Rarely	Rarely	Moderate	Most days
Starchy veg	Rarely	Occasionally	Most meals	Most days
Fruit	Every day	Twice a week	Small portions up to twice daily	At least 2 portions daily
Non-starchy veg	Every meal – lots of variety	Every meal – lots of variety	Every meal – lots of variety	Every meal – lots of variety
Nuts and seeds	Every day	Every day	Often	Often
Treats	Once a day	Dark chocolate every day	Dark chocolate. Almond muffins	Good-quality ice cream or dark chocolate
Alcohol	Twice a week	Most days	Twice a week max	A glass of wine a week
Drinks	Coffee, water	Coffee, water, chai	Water, coffee, redbush tea	Water, coffee

Identifying Your Health Goals

The beauty of the CarbScale approach is that it allows you to personalize your eating plan to meet your own health goals.

The table above illustrates the differing approaches of our team. All of us eat below 130g (4½oz) carbs a day and enjoy a varied and plentiful diet (remember current official guidelines encourage us to eat at least 250g (9oz) carbs a day!), with Giancarlo the strictest, and personal trainer Natalia the most carb-heavy. Katie and Jenny will flex their carb intake at the 75–100g (2¾–3½oz) mark, depending on exercise levels, how they feel, and what the scales say…

Tracking your carb intake is not difficult. This can be done easily by following the recipes in this book, checking the carb values of popular foods on pages 204–205 or looking at a guide such as *Carbs & Cals* (available as a book or as an app, which tracks your daily carb intake using a smart phone). However, you will be pleased to know that you don't need to become obsessed with counting carbs forever! You'll find that once you are following a low-carb way of living, it becomes natural not to go overboard.

The first step is to eliminate the main starchy offenders by finding delicious alternatives. The purpose of this book is to show you how. You can then make adjustments to meet your health goals.

Don't feel cheated – opposite are some delicious low-carb swaps you can make using this cookbook.

HIGH *carbs*

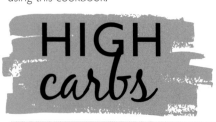
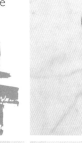
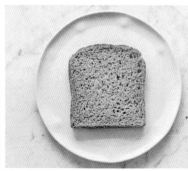

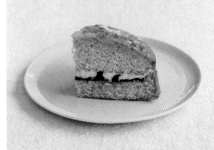
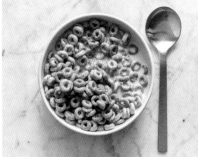
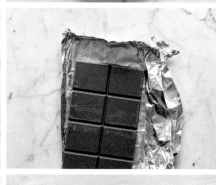

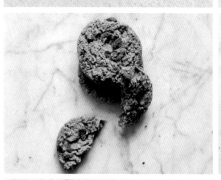
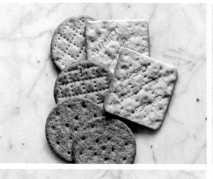
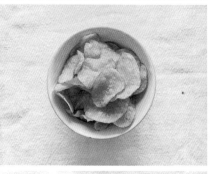

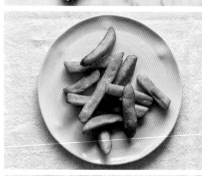
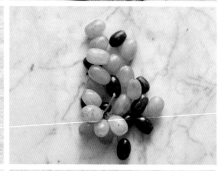
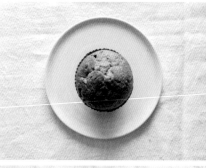

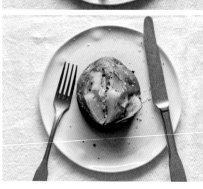
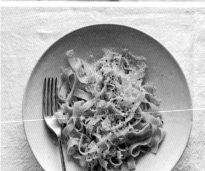
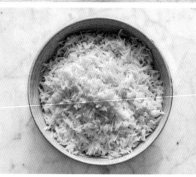

LOW carbs

Red wine

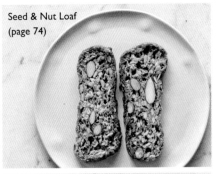

Seed & Nut Loaf
(page 74)

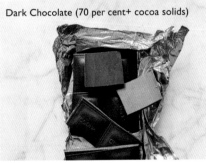

Peanut Butter & Jelly Cake
(page 186)

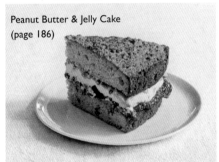

Cinnamon Granola
(page 60)

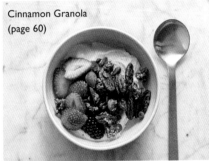

Dark Chocolate (70 per cent+ cocoa solids)

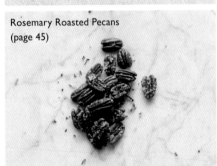

Rosemary Roasted Pecans
(page 45)

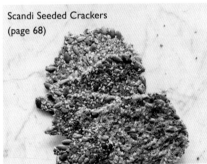

Scandi Seeded Crackers
(page 68)

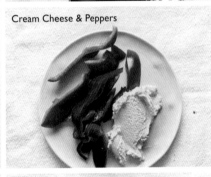

Cream Cheese & Peppers

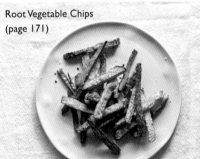

Root Vegetable Chips
(page 171)

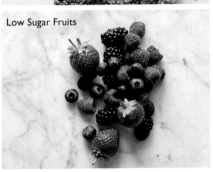

Low Sugar Fruits

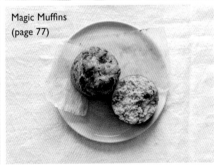

Magic Muffins
(page 77)

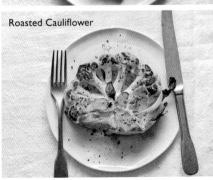

Roasted Cauliflower

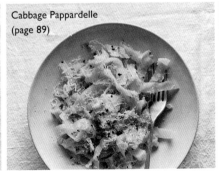

Cabbage Pappardelle
(page 89)

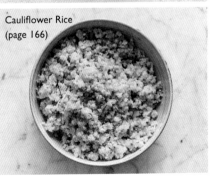

Cauliflower Rice
(page 166)

How Often Should You Eat?

'Eat little and often' is a mantra that many of us abide by, but if you have type 2 diabetes or want to lose weight this is not helpful advice. Every time you eat, digestive hormones and insulin are produced, which means your system just doesn't get a break.

Conversely, having breaks between meals, known as "intermittent fasting", can have many health benefits. When you are fasting your digestive system gets a rest and your body can concentrate on other vital jobs, such as keeping your immune system strong, balancing hormones and spring cleaning (detoxification!). It also helps to reduce and reset your insulin levels.

Try to aim for three meals a day without snacking in between – just like generations 50–60 years ago would have done. Once you get used to this, you should be able to go 5–6 hours between meals without feeling hungry.

If your goal is to lose weight, you may wish to experiment with even longer periods of intermittent fasting. Between meals, when insulin levels are low, you burn body fat which means you feel great and don't have dips in energy.

Eat only when you are hungry and not when convention tells you to or out of habit. Ask yourself if you really want that meal. If you don't feel you need breakfast, for example, then don't eat it. Contrary to popular belief, or as cereal manufacturers might like us to believe, breakfast is not necessarily the most important meal of the day.

Taking the idea of fasting further, you could try leaving 24 hours between meals once a week; fast between supper on day 1 and break it at supper on day 2. You might be surprised at how empowering it feels, and there are often knock-on effects in that your appetite becomes more controlled.

You may struggle at first with your perception of hunger between meals. However you will soon adjust and once your body can switch into fat-burning mode, burning calories from stored fat, it becomes easy to maintain gaps between meals. Instead of grabbing a snack, have a glass of water or a hot drink and focus on how much you will enjoy the next meal.

The graph below demonstrates that having frequent meals and snacks increases insulin levels and reduces the amount of time that the body is able to burn fat for energy.

THREE MEALS A DAY WITH REGULAR SNACKING

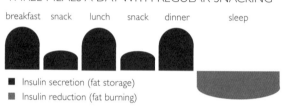

If someone is able to just consume three regular meals, there is more time over a 24 hour period where they are able to burn their stored body fat for energy.

THREE MEALS A DAY

Whereas, consuming just 1 or 2 meals per day vastly increases the fat-burning opportunity

INTERMITTENT FASTING

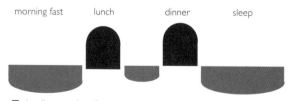

Diagram is reproduced with permission of Dr Trudi Deakin
www.xperthealth.org.uk

What to Expect in the First Few Days

When your carbohydrate intake is reduced, as it is when you switch to a low-carb diet, more of your energy is provided from fat. This is a perfectly normal process, and once you have adapted, you should find that your cravings for sweet and starchy foods are reduced, and that you feel more energized. In the first few days though, while your body adjusts, you may feel slightly light-headed and woozy, particularly when standing up from a sitting position.

The reason for this is that high insulin levels retain sodium via the kidneys. Once your insulin levels drop, then initially you lose both sodium and water; subsequently you may take more frequent trips to the bathroom. Drink more water to counter this, and add a sprinkle of natural salt (Himalayan, rock or sea salt) to your food.

The loss of sodium can also reduce your blood pressure naturally. If you are on hypertensive medication it may be a good idea to monitor your blood pressure. This sometimes has to be adjusted by your healthcare practitioner and so it is essential to discuss any dietary changes with them in advance.

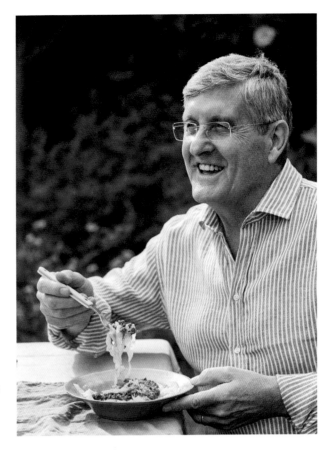

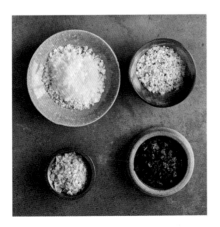

"I've never really wanted breakfast but was always told I should have it. Now I understand my blood sugar levels are high in the morning, so the last thing I need is breakfast, particularly a sugary one." Giancarlo

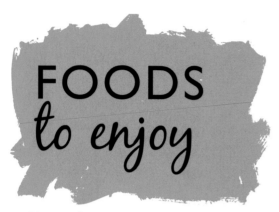

FOODS
to enjoy

You are about to embark on an abundant way of eating which is both delicious and satisfying. This section explores the three major food groups – protein, fats and carbs – and shows you how to construct meals which help to stabilize your blood sugar and nourish your body. By focusing on fresh ingredients, you will dramatically increase the quality of your food, which will pay off both in terms of your overall health and your energy levels.

Protein-rich Foods

Protein is a source of amino acids that are used in the growth and repair of our bodies. Just like a house is made of bricks, humans are primarily made of amino acids, some of which the body can make and others that have to be consumed within your diet.

We all need to eat good sources of protein – from animal foods and legumes to nuts, seeds, eggs and dairy. The amount of protein you require depends upon many factors, including your age, lifestyle and general health. For most of us a protein intake of 50–100g per day is usually about right (this is not the same as the fresh weight).

Vegetarians and vegans should consider their protein availability carefully and ensure that they have sufficient intake for good health; this is because vegetarian foods generally have a much lower protein density than animal products.

Protein content in popular foods

	Portion size	Protein content
Chicken breast	120g	38g
Salmon	120g	28g
Feta	75g	11g
Puy lentils	125g	12g
Tofu	100g	8g
Quinoa	50g	7g
Chickpeas	115g	8g
Sunflower seeds	30g	6g
Egg	One	8g
Walnuts	30g	4g
Broccoli	80g	4g
Kale	80g	3g

MEAT

Much as we love vegetables, there is no getting away from the fact that animal proteins are extremely nutritious. Meat is a rich source of easily digestible protein that makes it life-sustaining, and a great source of essential vitamins and minerals.

Meat, along with fish, is often the most expensive item in your shopping basket, but you don't need lots; a modest portion of 100–150g (3½–5oz) is plenty. Here are other ways to balance your budget:

● Buy whole joints, like a whole chicken, rather than individual pieces.
● Look for some of the cheaper cuts, like liver, which is just brimming with nutritional benefits, or stewing cuts.
● Meat coming to the end of its sell-by date will be discounted – buy and freeze this for another day.

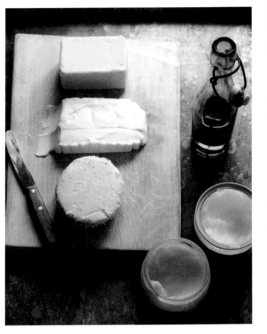

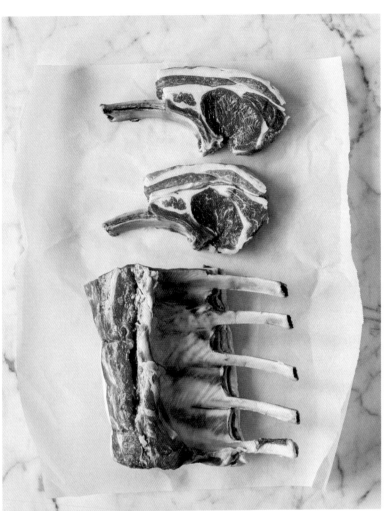

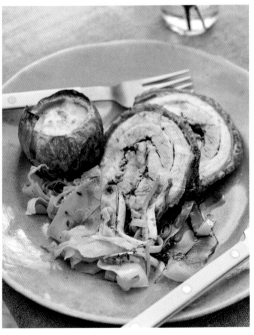

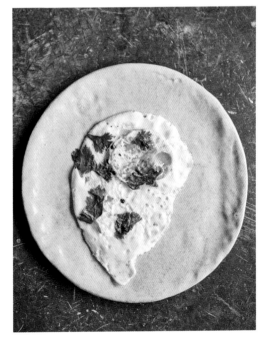

● Our local farm shop offers a 10 per cent discount on frozen meat, as it helps them to manage demand. Yours might do the same.

Try to vary the meat you enjoy. While there has been a trend towards consuming white meat like chicken, we strongly advocate red meat, too, which is delicious and nutritious. The World Health Organization suggests that up to 500g red meat per week is perfectly safe, which equates to three to four portions per week.

FISH

Fish is a fantastic source of protein and also has the benefit of being particularly quick to prepare. For example, the Super Quick Asian Salmon (page 132) takes only 15–20 minutes to cook and requires minimal preparation.

Oily fish is so called because it is rich in omega-3 essential fatty acids which are crucial for brain health and the nervous system (hence fish also has a mention in the fats and oils section opposite). Try to eat oily fish, such as salmon, mackerel, anchovies, sardines, trout and herring, at least twice a week

Non-oily fish, such as cod and seabass, can also be enjoyed regularly and takes on flavours very easily.

Keeping fish in the freezer means you have a ready supply on hand; simply put it in the fridge to defrost overnight. There is no nutritional difference between fish that has been frozen or canned as soon as it is caught and fresh fish, but steer clear of fish in breadcrumbs, as this adds unnecessary carbohydrate.

EGGS

Eggs are nature's wonder food – widely available, economical and extremely nutritious. Although they can be eaten at any time of day, eggs are often the star of a low-carb breakfast and we have several recipes for the mornings, from Courgette, Broccoli & Halloumi Scramble (page 59) to Smoked Salmon & Dill Breakfast Eggs (page 60).

Do not be afraid that eggs might raise your cholesterol levels. Since 2000, the Department of Health and the British Heart Foundation have changed their advice and removed limits to weekly egg consumption, as long as you eat a varied diet. Eggs are good for both brain and heart health.

DAIRY

Dairy contains both protein and fat. Hard cheeses, such as Parmesan, have one of the highest protein contents – 35g per 100g compared to 16g in feta. That said, the strong flavour of Parmesan lends itself more to an addition to a recipe, whereas feta may be the main event, such as in our Bouyiourdi (page 158).

Yogurt is a very popular food, though opt for a natural full-fat version and add your own fruit like berries. Low-fat fruit-flavoured yogurts can contain up to three times as much carbohydrate compared to full-fat Greek yogurt.

Dairy is also a good source of calcium and vitamin D which helps to make bones strong. In the past, you may have restricted cheese and other dairy products due to their fat content. The good news is that higher fat foods can actually contribute to health and weight loss provided that you are keeping your carbohydrate intake low… more about that shortly (see opposite).

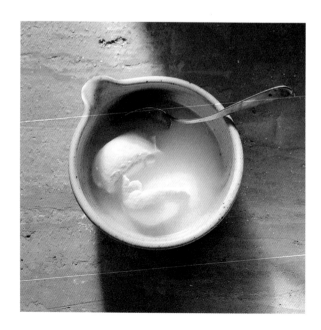

PULSES

This food group includes beans and lentils, which are high in fibre and extremely economical. Pulses are particularly useful in Asian dishes, where they take on flavours beautifully. They are moderately high in carbs, so our recipes mix them with vegetables to reduce the spike in blood sugar that they may otherwise cause. Where pulses are added to dishes, such as A Great Greek Salad (page 154), they can bulk up a recipe, making it go further.

How frequently you enjoy pulses does depend on what your health goals are, and where you are on the CarbScale. If you are on a strict programme and are striving to get your blood sugars under control, then they are best avoided until your blood sugar levels have stabilized.

Fats and Oils

If you have had a past history of regular dieting you are probably familiar with fat avoidance.

Fat has been picked on as a dietary culprit because it contains more calories per gram than either protein or carbohydrate. But healthy fats, from natural sources, are an essential part of a low-carb diet. In fact, it can be easier to manage your total calorie intake with a higher fat diet, and this can help weight loss and improving metabolic health.

There are two good reasons for this:

1. Fat doesn't drive your blood sugar or insulin levels upwards, which keeps your fat storage in check.
2. Eating more fat helps to stabilize your appetite, so that you can eat less and feel less hungry.

There is no need to be concerned about natural fats (including saturated fats) contributing to heart disease. The PURE study assessed the dietary intake of over 135,000 individuals across 18 countries and followed them for seven years. The study found that carbohydrate intake was linked with higher mortality, and fat intake was associated with both lower mortality and lower risk of cardiac events. Astonishingly, saturated fat had an inverse relationship with stroke –

> "The joy of a low-carb diet is that foods which you may have avoided for decades can now be enjoyed."

this means that the higher the saturated fat intake the lower the stroke risk. A further study suggests that full-fat dairy products may reduce the risk of death from cardiovascular disease.

The joy of a low-carb diet is that foods which you may have avoided for decades can now be enjoyed. Avocado, cream and butter are all on the menu, along with nuts, seeds and fatty (and tasty!) meat and fish. You can also use speciality oils in salads for extra taste, such as avocado, walnut or sesame seed oils. Just bear in mind, if you want to lose weight, then limit or even avoid snacking on good fats, as you really want to burn your own body fat for energy between meals.

In addition to cooking with butter or ghee, you can use olive oil and coconut oil. We love old-fashioned animal fats, like tallow and lard, which can be collected from roasting a joint. This reduces waste and makes food really tasty, something that makes the low-carb lifestyle effective in the long term; the food is so enjoyable that you will not want to go back to your old ways.

However, a word of caution: all fats are not equal and we recommend that industrially-processed vegetable oils, such as corn and sunflower oil, and margarines should be avoided. Though often advertised as 'heart-friendly', these oils are unstable when heated, producing toxic aldehydes that are prone to damage cells and cause inflammation. In an Australian study of men who had suffered a recent heart attack, those consuming margarines in place of saturated fats like butter had increased rates of heart and cardiovascular disease. It is now generally regarded that the case against butter has been misguided, resulting in headlines like 'butter is back'.

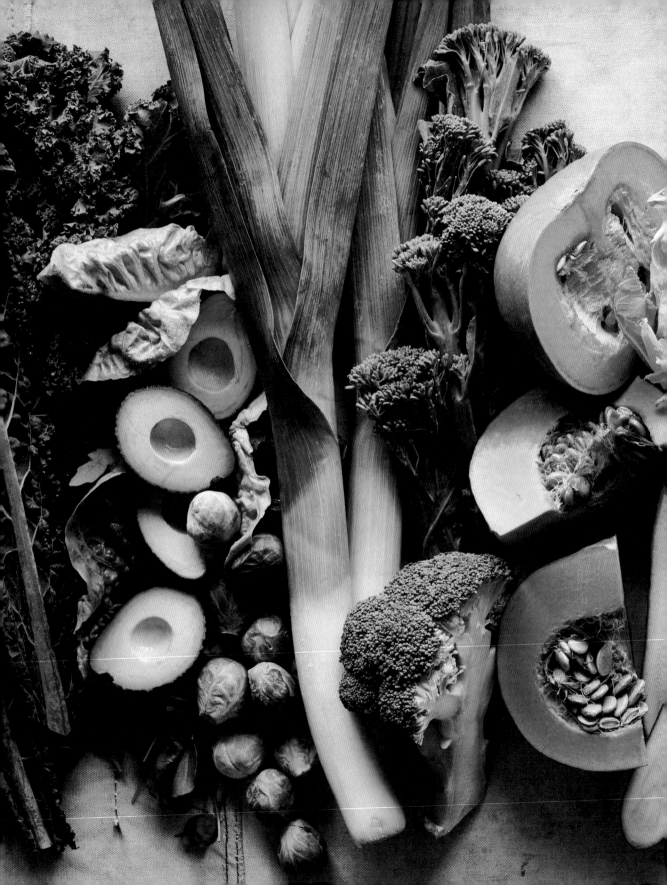

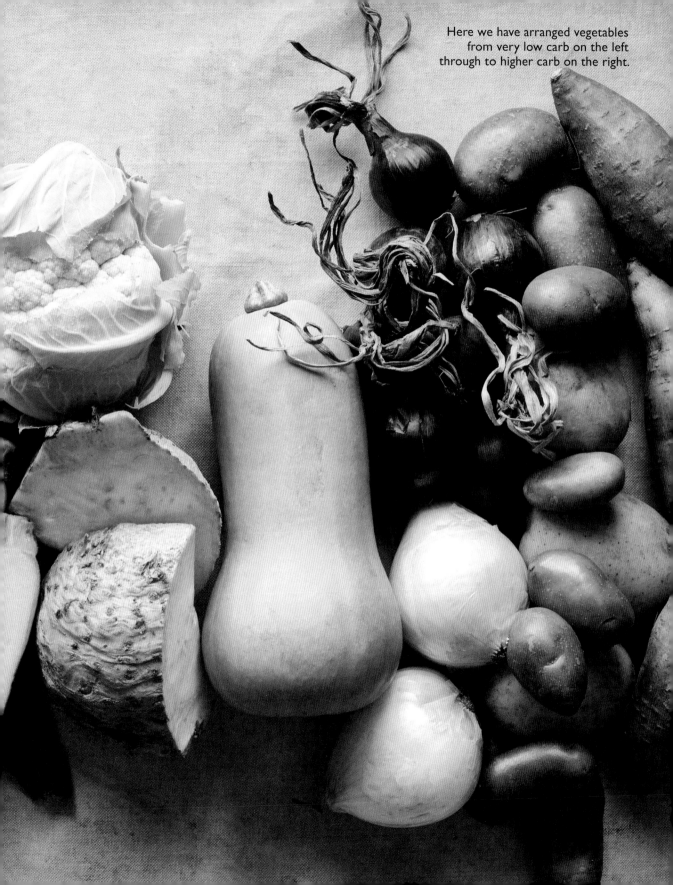

Here we have arranged vegetables from very low carb on the left through to higher carb on the right.

Carbohydrates

The extent to which you choose to limit your starchy or higher carbohydrate foods depends on your own health goals. Go lower for weight loss or blood sugar control, and be more relaxed if you are lean, active and healthy. Our recipes will help to guide you, by making meal suggestions and also including the nutritional values of the dish so that you can experiment with how much carbohydrate you can tolerate. You can also look up the carb value of popular foods in the Appendix (pages 204–205).

Carbohydrate-rich foods include vegetables (which everyone should eat), fruit and grains. Protein-rich foods, such as pulses and quinoa, also have a significant carbohydrate content so make sure you are aware of this when you are eating according to the CarbScale. If your blood sugars remain too high, then you may need to avoid them.

VEGETABLES

Bring on the veg – they add bulk to your recipes and help to fill you up; they increase variety at mealtimes, with so many different types to choose from; they also pack a punch in terms of nutrients, consistently adding vitamins and minerals to your diet, which are essential for your body's metabolism.

Increasing your vegetable intake is a fabulous investment in your health, and it can really help in your quest to reduce starchy carbs like bread, potatoes, rice and pasta. Simply increase the number of vegetables to compensate for the starchy carbs that you used to eat. This allows you to easily adjust your diet alongside family mealtimes, with only small tweaks when others might not need to, or want to, cut their own carb portions.

We differentiate between non-starchy and starchy vegetables; the latter includes root vegetables which grow underground and concentrate sugars for storage, resulting in a higher glycaemic index (GI). These can be eaten in restricted amounts, whereas non-starchy vegetables can be eaten freely.

FRUIT

Although fruit is good for you, especially compared to refined and processed foods, it is still naturally

NON-STARCHY VEGETABLES

Non-starchy vegetables are listed in the food plan (see page 23), and include:

- green leafy and salad vegetables
- the cruciferous family (broccoli, cauliflower, kale)
- the allium family (onions, garlic)
- Mediterranean vegetables (peppers, aubergines, courgettes)
- asparagus
- mushrooms
- green beans
- celeriac
- fennel
- artichoke

STARCHY VEGETABLES (LIMIT PORTIONS)

- butternut squash
- parsnips
- carrots
- beetroot
- sweet potatoes
- pumpkin
- turnip
- swede

quite sugary and so can raise your blood sugar levels. Generally, berries are very low sugar and can be enjoyed even if you are on a strict low-carb plan.

Sometimes we use fruit within a recipe because it adds a touch of luxury and enjoyment to the meal. The overall carb content can be contained because it is mixed with other ingredients, such as the Cinnamon Granola (page 60), which uses a very small amount of dates.

We have also used fruit as a natural sweetener in baking, such as the apple or pear in the Magic Muffins (page 77). Baked goods tend to be high in calories, so please view them as an occasional treat rather than an everyday indulgence.

Be very careful with the amount of fruit you include in smoothies, as these can be extremely high in sugar.

Low-sugar fruit: berries and cherries
Medium-sugar fruit: apples, pears, peaches, nectarines, plums
Higher-sugar fruit: tropical fruits, such as banana, melon, pomegranate, mango and pineapple, and dried fruits

GRAINS

Some 10,000 years ago, we made the transition from hunter-gatherers to farmers – this was the agricultural revolution. It enabled humans to settle in villages, and was made possible due to the cultivation of grain – wheat, rice, corn, millet, barley – and potatoes.

Farming did enable the human population to expand rapidly, as the food supply could be managed, but there were downsides. Yuval Noah Harari points out in his excellent book, *Sapiens: A Brief History of Humankind*: "A diet based on cereals is poor in vitamins and minerals, hard to digest and really bad for your teeth and gums." Quite a dietary insight from an anthropologist! Add to this the disruptive blood sugar effects when grain and cereal are overeaten, and you can see why the modern diet – up to 55 per cent of calories based on these foods – is a disaster.

There is one grain-based recipe included in this book – the Ham Hock & Pea Risotto (page 93), where we have combined farro with vegetables to reduce the effect on blood sugar levels and increase nutrients. This offers some variety if you don't need to be quite so strict – it really depends on how well-managed your blood sugar levels are.

If you are lean and healthy, you may be able to indulge occasionally, and in moderation, in some good-quality artisan bread like sourdough, which is more digestible due to the slow fermentation process. But we also give a very tasty low-carb bread recipe for Baguettes or brown rolls using psyllium husk powder (a type a fibre) on page 69.

The Caldesi family, being Italian, do love pasta! However, Giancarlo rarely, if ever, indulges even in gluten-free pasta, while Katie enjoys her favourite bowl of pasta and ragù every now and then. A low-carb option we all love is a creamy tomato sauce over some roasted vegetables (see page 90).

Treats

Who doesn't love the occasional treat or celebration? Food is almost always a part of major life events – from birthdays and weddings, to just socializing with friends. However, what was once a treat for a special occasion has now become part of everyday life, and we are consuming too much sweet and sugary stuff.

As you begin to include more fresh foods within your diet, we hope that your palate begins to change – you may even find that the naughty foods which you used to crave are no longer quite so enjoyable.

We are not killjoys and do recognize that you still want to have some fun around food, hence the healthier versions of popular treats like our low-carb Hot Chocolate Pots (page 184) and a range of mini puds to finish off a special meal (see pages 182–195).

It is worth pointing out that a couple of squares of very dark chocolate (70–85 per cent cocoa solids) can also be enjoyed occasionally. Dark chocolate has relatively low sugar levels and is also a source of magnesium and antioxidants.

Alcohol is considered a treat; after all, you don't drink it because you are thirsty! Beer, lager and cider are out if you are watching your blood sugar levels – they contain up to 18g carbs (or 4½ teaspoons sugar) per pint, which explains the beer belly! Wine is a better choice but keep within the guidelines of 14 units per week – this equates to around six 175ml glasses. Red wine may have slightly more positive health benefits due to its resveratrol content; this is an antioxidant which helps to protect cells from damage.

"A treat is once a week, but if it becomes once a day, it is no longer a treat."
Dr David Unwin

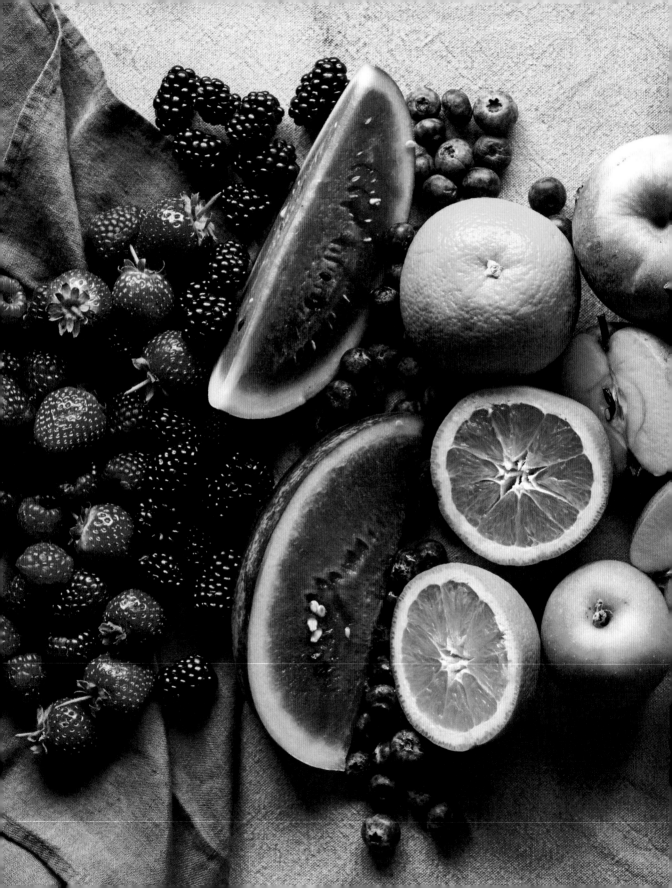

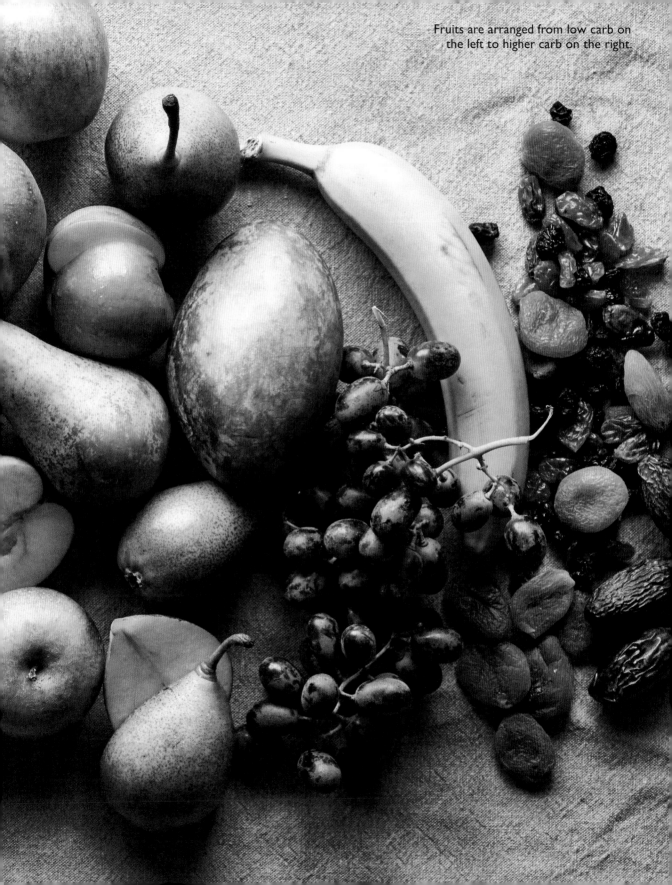

Fruits are arranged from low carb on the left to higher carb on the right.

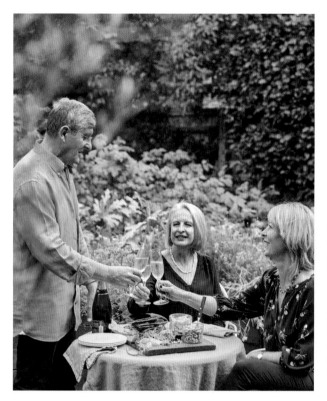

Beware of the hidden sugars in drinks sold at high street coffee shops. If you enjoy coffee, then a good choice is an Americano or filter coffee, either black or with full-fat milk or cream. This may sound surprising but it is carbs that you are restricting not fats; many people report that adding cream is satiating and helps them to control their appetite. Don't add a syrupy shot to your coffee – this is pure sugar and will send your insulin levels soaring.

Obviously as this is a low-sugar plan, sweet squash, juices, cordials and sodas are completely out, and this includes the diet varieties. Whether based on artificial sweeteners or sugar, these drinks will likely fuel food cravings for the wrong foods, and hence contribute to weight gain either directly or indirectly.

Do be aware, though, that alcohol is a significant source of calories: one 175ml glass of wine clocks up to 190 calories, which may later sit around your waistline.

Drinks

Your number one health-giving drink is… water. Enjoy it still or sparkling, add a slice of lemon or lime, or maybe even try it warm between meals, particularly if you are trying to reduce your snacking. Often when you get cravings for food, it can be a sign that you are dehydrated, so always drink water or a hot or cold drink before reaching for a snack.

Regular tea and coffee is also allowed on the CarbScale plan, but just check how many cups you are drinking in a day. If you are drinking multiple cups to give yourself a little caffeine hit, then this might be a sign that you need to cut your intake. Some people find the caffeine in regular tea and coffee makes them jittery, which is also a sign to decrease consumption. We list hot and cold drink alternatives on pages 196–203.

YOUR FOOD PLAN
Using the food plan opposite, according to where you are on the CarbScale, is a helpful tool to manage your carb intake. These nutritious ingredients are used within the recipes in this book. Many commercially produced foods are very high-carb so always check the label and pay attention to the total carbs per serving, not just the sugars.

Your Food Plan

LOW CARB – eat freely	MEDIUM CARB – go easy	HIGH CARB – caution!
Meat and fish: Beef, chicken, duck, lamb, pork, turkey, venison. High quality sausages (97% meat) and bacon. All types of fish including seafood e.g. prawns		
Veg: Asparagus, aubergine, avocado, broccoli, Brussels sprouts, cabbage, cauliflower, celeriac, celery, courgettes, cucumbers, fennel, green beans, kale, leeks, mushrooms, olives, onions, peas, peppers, pumpkin, rocket, salad greens, spinach, string beans, tomatoes, watercress	Beetroot, butternut squash, carrots, parsnip, swede, sweetcorn, turnip	Potato, sweet potato
Nuts and seeds: Almond, chestnut, hazelnut, macadamia, pecan, pistachio, walnut, peanut. Chia, flax, pumpkin, sesame, sunflower seeds	Cashew	
Fats and oils: Animal fats e.g. goose or duck fat, butter, coconut oil, lard, olive oil. Speciality oils eg: sesame. Mayonnaise.		
Eggs and dairy: Eggs, natural or Greek full-fat yogurt, cream, cheese	Milk	
Pulses: None	Black-eyed beans, chickpeas, lentils, etc.	
Fruit: Berries: all types, cherries, lemon, lime	Apple (eaten as the whole fruit and not juice), apricot, nectarine, peach, pear, plum	Banana and dried fruit (unless used in small amounts), grapes, orange, satsuma, tropical fruits
Beverages: Unsweetened herbal teas. Green tea. Water, still or sparkling. Bone broth	Red wine, dry white wine (including champagne) – in moderation!	Beer, cider
Grains and flours: None		Oats, rice, pasta, quinoa, flours – gram, buckwheat, rye, spelt, wheat
Treats: Refer to this cookbook for low-carb treats – substitute nut flours for healthy baking	70%+ cocoa solids dark chocolate	

Mind Over Matter:
How Thoughts Can Help or Hinder Your Plans

Dr Jen Unwin is a psychologist within the NHS and has been involved with running low-carb patient groups. With her specialist skills, she can help to address some of the emotional and mental barriers which are involved in any change to your regular behaviours and habits, such as what you eat!

"Cutting out carbs and sugar means I don't need to constantly count calories or be yo-yo dieting. My energy levels, skin and hair are all better. I no longer eat breakfast and can happily go until lunchtime. I can still cook for the family, too."

HERE ARE JEN'S TOP TIPS FOR MAXIMUM MOTIVATION:

1 **Before you start, have a think** about why you are hoping to make changes to your way of eating. What are you hoping for? To come off medication? To feel better? To lose weight? To stay active and healthy longer? If you have a good reason for making changes and are aware of hoped-for outcomes, it will spur you on. What difference would it make to you if you could achieve your goals?

2 **We all overestimate willpower.** It wanes after a few weeks, and we are all susceptible to 'lapse' when we are tired or stressed. Maximize your chances of success by advance planning and making changes to your environment. Out of sight is definitely out of mind. If you can, clear out your cupboards of foods you don't want to eat before you start. If you need to keep starchy food in the house for other family members, then put it on a separate shelf and buy it in portioned packages, such as bags of microwaveable rice, so you are not tempted to 'just have a bit' when you cook it for someone else.

3 Sugar and carbohydrates give us a "feel-good factor" due to the effect they have on the brain and the way they help to release "happy hormones". Try to think of other, non-food, mood boosts. Take a walk; start, or re-start a creative hobby; do some volunteering; or plan outings with friends and family. Make these a regular part of your week.

4 **We are essentially social animals** so it's a good idea to link in with other people on the same journey. There are lots of social media communities, such as www.diabetes.co.uk/lowcarbforum, where you can ask questions and celebrate your successes. Also, if you are going to increase your activity levels, it could be a good motivator to do that with a friend or family member.

5 While you may have a big goal, such as losing a certain amount of weight, it's also important to notice and enjoy little victories, such as someone complimenting you, your trousers feeling looser or going a week without a biscuit!

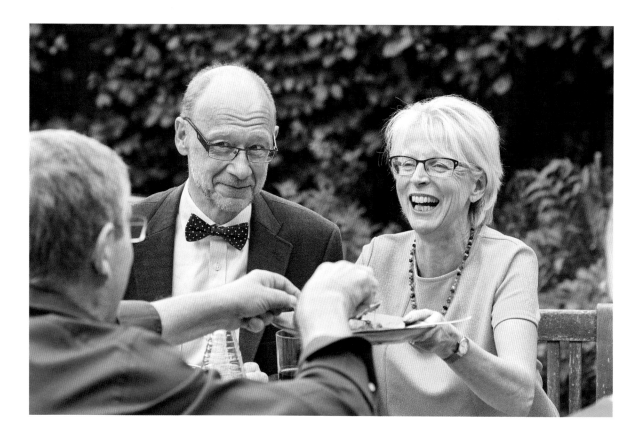

6 You will overeat or eat the wrong things from time to time. Use these wobbles as a chance to reflect on why they happened and how you might avoid the pitfalls next time. Get straight back into your routine without too much self-criticism.

7 Be honest. If you are finding it hard to change your diet? Might you actually be a "sugar addict"? Do you struggle to just have one biscuit? Do you crave sugar and find it difficult to cut down, despite wanting to and knowing it is harming you? It can be a real battle to give up something you love even if you know it is doing you harm. Sugar is very addictive, so cutting down is hard. You have two main ways to tackle this. Some people are better slowly cutting down sugar and carbs and swapping foods for low-sugar/lower carb options: bread for oatcakes, cereal for yogurt, fruit and nuts, etc. Some people will never manage this graduated approach (a bit like a person with an alcohol addiction can never just have one drink). The solution in that case may be "cold turkey". Pick a day and give up sugar and carbs. Make sure you plan and also be prepared for a tough few days at the start. Believe me, after a week or so you will feel amazing. Have plenty of water and a little extra salt to avoid headaches and fatigue.

8 The long-term goal is to eat less often, snack less and eat real, fresh food. You may need smaller steps to get you there. For example, allow yourself a mid-afternoon snack at first. The important thing is that you learn from your own experience. We are all unique and have to fit the principles around what suits us and our families. This is why we don't give exact amounts to follow. You need to learn what works for you.

"It's a mindset. This is more than a diet; this is a way of life."
Giancarlo

Will This Plan Really Work For Me?

Making changes to your eating habits is a really big deal. We spend a lot of time both thinking about and preparing food. So is it worth it? It certainly is if you are looking to make a step change in your health. We share the results here to help give you the confidence that it really could work for you too.

Jenny has been using this low-carb eating plan with clients for over ten years and the results are amazing, not just in terms of weight management, but in how people look and feel. Dr Unwin measures clinical improvements and you may find his results really inspiring. And, of course, Katie and Giancarlo have first-hand experience of Giancarlo's journey back to health.

The table below shows the improvements in Dr Unwin's patient group, all of whom were diagnosed with type 2 diabetes. Key highlights are:

Significant weight loss – on average this patient group lost 8.9kg (nearly 20lb)!

Cardiovascular health improves – cholesterol, triglycerides or fats in the blood and blood pressure all improve. Dr Unwin is able to reduce hypertensive medication for around a third of his patients when they go "low carb".

Blood sugar control improves – HbA1c decreases and nearly 1 in 4 reverse their type 2 diabetes.

Liver function improves – Gamma GT, a marker which is raised when the liver becomes fatty, decreases.

THE WIDER PICTURE

In addition, the excellent results of a low-carb approach have now been verified by research. A recently published paper evaluating the one-year outcomes of the online Low-Carb Program produced by Diabetes.co.uk for people with type 2 diabetes showed an impressive average weight loss of 6.9 per cent of participant's body weight. Of the participants who were taking at least one drug for their diabetes at the start, an amazing 40 per cent were able to reduce one or more of their medications – and yet still show significantly improved control of diabetes.

Another study compared the metabolic rate of people on diets containing 20 per cent, 40 per cent and 60 per cent carbs (where all food was provided over the study period). Those eating the lowest carb diet burned about 250 calories a day more than those eating the most carbs. This likely explains why people report feeling very well on a low-carb diet, as they are using their calories to make energy.

> "I thought, what have I got to lose? Going low carb has changed my life." Jenny

Dr Unwin's clinical results – 86 patients over 20 months																	
	HbA1c			Total cholesterol			HDL cholesterol			Cholesterol ratio			Triglyceride					
Averages	Start	Finish	Loss	Start	Finish	Loss	Start	Finish	Loss	Start	Finish	Loss	Start	Finish	Loss			
	67.9	47.2	**20.7**	4.9	4.4	**0.5**	1.29	1.46	**-0.17**	4.3	3.8	**0.5**	2.54	1.65	**0.89**			
This includes 21 cases of full T2D remission a rate of 24%	Weight in kg			Systolic BP in mmHg			Diastolic BP in mmHb			Gamma-G.T level in U/L								
	Start	Finish	Loss	Start	Finish	Loss	Start	Finish	Loss	Start	Finish	Loss						
	98.1	89.2	**8.9**	143	134	**9**	86	78	**8**	79.9	43.0	36.9						

Getting Started

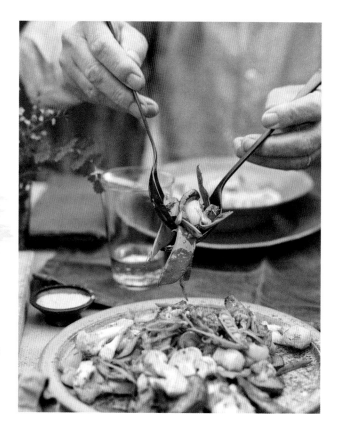

If you are on medication, make an appointment to discuss your plans with your medical professional so that they can monitor and revise your prescription as required.

KEEP A FOOD DIARY

It really helps to write down everything that passes your lips, and then to reflect on it – can you see patterns? Which are your best meals? With the knowledge you are now gaining, which meals or snacks are not helping? Where could you start to make changes? Knowledge is power.

If you don't like to write things down, then take a picture of what you eat – absolutely everything! We underestimate what we eat all the time.

The more honest you are with yourself, the easier you will find it to start making changes and seeing results.

WRITE DOWN YOUR GOALS

Be clear on what you would like to achieve. The more visual you can make this the more compelling it can be. Reflect on Dr Jen Unwin's tips on pages 40–41.

How will you assess your results? Have a process for reviewing and revising your plan so that you move closer to your goal.

TRANSITION ONE MEAL AT A TIME

It can be overwhelming to change all of your food habits at once. Try focusing on just one mealtime: breakfast, lunch or dinner. Choose three recipes from this category and decide when you will try them out. If you enjoy them and they fit in with your lifestyle, then make those recipes a regular thing so you are widening your repertoire. If they don't suit you, move on and try a different recipe.

Once you have mastered one mealtime, choose another. In no time, you will have transitioned into a new way of eating.

BE PREPARED!

You know it makes sense… plan, shop and prepare in a way that works for you. Jenny prefers to prep in the morning so she has food in the fridge ready to go. Often she'll use a slow cooker, so all she needs to do is steam vegetables at the end of the day. Katie, on the other hand, loves to cook in the evening with the kids and often uses a pressure cooker to speed things up.

Try batch-cooking and freezing the meal in portions so you know that you always have something you can defrost that is low-carb.

AVOID TEMPTATION

Buy in all the lovely food and ingredients you can eat and ensure they are accessible. Online shopping is brilliant if you are prone to temptation in the supermarket; make a list and get your staples delivered straight to your door. When you do go shopping, it is a good idea not to venture out when you are hungry for. Depending on your family's needs it may help to clear your cupboards of foods that are 'off plan' for you.

MAKE TIME

If you are juggling work and feel pressed for time, try to keep things simple. Refer to the Quick and Easy Snack ideas on page 45 for inspiration.

Perhaps try reframing your view of cooking to become a hobby rather than a chore. Could your partner or family become involved, so you can have quality time together as you chop, mix and cook? A traditional Italian family is a role model for this style of living – the kitchen is the heart of family life.

TAKE TIME

Do you rush your meals, shovelling down mouthfuls while sitting in front of the TV? Or do you find yourself mindlessly snacking? Both can lead to overeating and increase the risk of weight gain.

Try to make a point of focusing your attention at mealtimes, preferably sitting at a table and even better in company so you can chat while you eat. Take your time, maybe putting down your cutlery between bites and appreciating the flavours, rather than wolfing it down.

Another top tip is to split meals into courses, which is very European. Being Italian, Giancarlo often starts with a fresh salad rather than having it with his main course. Or you could have a small bowl of soup as a starter. It's not about eating more, but spreading out your meal with courses to help your body recognize when you are full.

EATING OUT AND TAKEAWAYS

We are frequently told that people find low-carb eating to be a lot easier to manage in restaurants than calorie counting. You are looking to fill up on good-quality protein and vegetables, so don't be afraid to ask for slight variations to the menu, such as ordering two starters rather than a main course, or requesting extra salad in place of chips.

You may also think about asking for the bread basket to be removed, as this can set off a wave of carby cravings. Instead, opt for olives to snack on, or drink more water to distract yourself until the food arrives.

Puddings can be a bit hairy on the sugar front, so choose a coffee to finish your meal, or order some fresh fruit (preferably berries) with fresh cream or a cheese course (just leave those carby crackers alone).

If the occasional takeaway is your guilty pleasure, try to reduce the overall carbs in your order. Have a curry,

but not the rice or naan bread; have a kebab, but not the pitta; have a burger, but not the bun. Try asking for extra salad and low-carb vegetable dishes to bulk out your meal. Alternatively, in the time it takes to have a curry or Chinese delivered, make your own Cauliflower Rice (page 166) or Green Stir-Fry (page 172).

SMART SERVINGS

Because you no longer have rice or mash to mop up sauces, you may find serving meals in a bowl with a spoon and fork an easier way to enjoy this new way of eating.

Reduce your portion sizes. Don't put the food on the table as this makes it too easy to have seconds. Serve up by the hob and take the plates to the table. Many of us still have a "no waste" mentality so we eat everything on our plates; you don't need to finish everything. Leave it until tomorrow and make another meal from it.

Reduce your plate size – according to Cornell University Food and Brand Lab, this can help you eat 30 per cent less food.

FOOD ON THE GO

- Walnut and Parmesan Seeded Rolls (page 70) filled with cooked chicken and mayo
- Quick Smoked Mackerel Pâté (page 128), vegetables, feta and olives
- Put any of the salads in a jar (pages 119, 122, 152, 153, 154), dressings taken separately or at the bottom of the jar
- David Unwins's microwave vegetables and leftovers (page 180)
- Magic Muffins (page 77)
- Wraps (page 81) with Tahini Sauce (page 144) and Italian Roasted Vegetables (page 144)
- Avocado, miniature bottle of dressing, teaspoon all in a bag – cut avocado but keep it together

SNACKS

If you are following intermittent fasting (see page 26), then snacks may not be for you. However, for some people they are part of a transition from high- to low-carb. In the past, David coped with his long surgery hours with a packet of biscuits in his drawer. Then he swapped to pecan nuts instead. Now he has no need for either. There may be times when you would prefer a healthy snack in preference to a meal or, like Natalia, you may have high activity levels.

Sometimes it is the ceremony of it – if you are used to opening a bag of peanuts or cheesy crisps with your partner over a glass of wine before dinner, then admit it. When Katie cooks she picks at the food at the same time. If that is your weak point, have some celery sticks or slices of red pepper to hand, but ban the crisps.

If all else fails, go to the fridge and get out what you want to snack on. Close the door of the fridge, prepare the food in the right quantity and put it onto a plate. Do not stand at the fridge with the door open eating – you simply won't know how much you have eaten! Sit at a table with a glass of water and mindfully enjoy your snack. Do not go back to the fridge for another helping. Step away from your plate, move out of the kitchen and do something else for 15 minutes; you will feel full enough. Go back to the kitchen later and wash up the plate feeling smug that you didn't overeat!

HERE ARE SOME QUICK AND EASY SNACK IDEAS:

- Scandi Seeded Crackers (page 68) with cream cheese and tomato
- Drinks such as Beef Bone Broth (page 112), Chai Tea (page 201) or coffee and cream
- A slice of chicken or turkey
- Olives
- Slices of red pepper with a dip
- Quick Smoked Mackerel Pâté (page 128) and celery sticks
- Boiled eggs
- Greek yogurt and a swirl of peanut butter
- Cold meats – Jenny rolls up ham with cream cheese
- Celery sticks and peanut butter
- Apple and peanut butter with cinnamon
- 25g nuts and seeds, but watch out for the dried fruit
- A whole punnet of berries with a little Greek yogurt or cream
- Small pre-wrapped squares of good-quality dark chocolate – over 85 per cent cocoa solids only
- 30g mixed cheese cubes, salted pecans and olives

ROSEMARY-ROASTED PECANS

On a long car journey with the Unwins, Jen treated us to these nuts, cheese and olives. Almonds, Brazil nuts, hazelnuts and macadamia nuts work well too. Serves 6
Preheat the oven to 200°C/fan 180°C/gas mark 6. Toss 200g pecans in a bowl with 2 tablespoons extra virgin olive oi, ½ teaspoon salt flakes and 1 tablespoon finely chopped rosemary. Pour onto a baking tray and flatten out into a single layer. Roast for 5–8 minutes or until lightly browned. Leave to cool to room temperature and serve. The nuts will keep well in container for up to a week.
Per serving: 1.9g carbs, 3.6g protein, 27g fat, 2.6g fibre, 273kcal

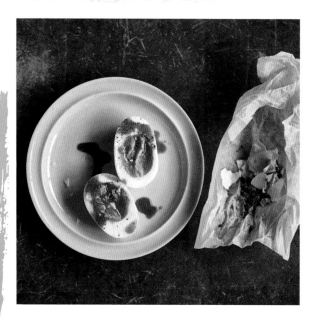

What to Do If Weight Loss Stalls

If you find that you hit a weight plateau, here are some tips to get you back into fat-burning mode:

● It's time for reflection. How closely are you sticking to your eating plan? Do you binge at the weekend – another glass of wine, some crisps, a slice of toast – and then work hard on denial during the week? It may feel like you're in full-on carb restriction, but the only way to really know is to keep a food diary and assess whether you truly are.
● Trust that the way to sustained weight loss is not through calorie counting. The chances are that you've been counting calories for many years, yet you're still not consistently at your goal weight. You need a new approach!
● If you've already made strides to reduce your sugar and starchy carb intake, have you gone far enough? The beauty of CarbScale is that you can adjust it to suit your own goals. Select some of the recipes which are lower carb and begin to add them to your repertoire.
● Have the snacks gone, especially those low-calorie (aka high-carb) ones? Intermittent fasting means eating nothing between meals – even a tiny bite will release insulin and put the brakes on your body's attempts to burn fat.
● How often are you drinking alcohol? The calories in booze will be burned instead of fat, and drinking alcohol also increases your appetite. If you regularly enjoy a glass of wine or two, now may be the time to try a short period of abstinence to see if that helps. It need not be forever. Try making some delicious alcohol-free drinks instead (see pages 198–203).
● Are you drinking enough water? Often when we think we are hungry, a large glass of tepid water can be a great distraction. Try to keep a jug or large bottle of water close by so that you can easily keep hydrated and monitor how much you're actually drinking per day.
● Find some time to de-stress. Cortisol, which is released in times of stress, is a catabolic hormone which can scupper your efforts to lose weight by breaking down muscle into glucose (this is called "gluconeogenesis" and occurs primarily in the liver). This helps to fuel you for "fight or flight" response, but losing muscle mass will reduce your metabolic rate and make you more likely to put on weight. So take up yoga, restructure your work day, assess your relationships, get more sleep… Do whatever it takes for you to feel more relaxed.
● Are you moving enough? In the next section, personal trainer Natalia will outline the benefits of exercise for overall health and weight loss.

> "Take up yoga, restructure your work day, assess your relationships, get more sleep … Do whatever it takes for you to feel more relaxed."

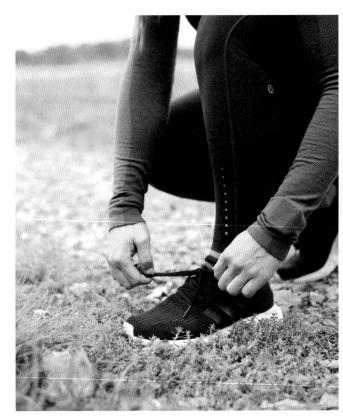

Movement

By Natalia Giers (www.strictlyfitpt.co.uk)

I qualified as a personal trainer exactly ten years ago. Since achieving my qualifications, fitness has become my full-time job and my passion. I feel very strongly about maintaining a healthy mind and body through a balanced lifestyle. I feel it's our responsibility to look after and educate ourselves on what is the best approach for us to achieve optimum health. Not everyone can become an athlete, but everyone can become fit by taking responsibility for their lifestyle. If there is a will there is always a way.

WHY IS IT IMPORTANT TO BE ACTIVE?
- Dr Unwin believes that people who exercise regularly look better and live longer.
- Exercise can aid weight loss.
- Exercise reduces blood pressure and makes heart disease and stroke less likely.
- Exercise can improve balance, which is important because many people with type 2 diabetes or obesity are at risk of falls.
- Activity boosts energy and lifts your mood.
- Exercise increases bone strength and density.
- A study carried out in 2008 showed that two hours of TV time a day is associated with a 20% increase in the risk of type 2 diabetes and that five hours gave a 50% increase.

Dietary changes are a great way of reducing your risk of diabetes and obesity, but let's not forget about the amazing and complementary benefits of movement. Humans are not a sedentary species – we are designed to be moving – yet in modern society it has become normal to move very little. In fact, we often make a conscious effort to move as little as possible: we drive to the corner shop, we park as near to the gym as possible (how ironic!) and we even take the lift to the first floor.

It's so important to do cardiovascular exercise because it enhances the ability of the heart and lungs to supply oxygen-rich blood to the working muscles and organs. In turn, this makes our bodies more efficient and increases our energy levels.

Weight training is also very beneficial because it increases lean muscle mass, which can boost your base metabolic rate and cause you to burn calories at a faster rate, even at rest. The ability of your muscles to use up glucose increases with your strength, making your body more efficient at regulating its blood sugar levels. So, as your body's muscle-to-fat ratio increases, the amount of insulin you need in your body to help store energy in fat cells reduces. From being insulin resistant you can train your body to be more insulin sensitive with exercise.

How to Become More Active

Getting fit can mean different things to different people and, to ensure steady improvement, here are some ideas on how to incorporate more movement into your daily routine:

- Change your attitude! Decide not to be a couch potato and start being more active. Dr Unwin gets up from his desk and goes to the waiting room to collect his patients instead of sitting down waiting for them. This means he moves every 10 minutes. What might be your first, small step towards being more active?
- Be realistic and set sensible goals. If you absolutely hate exercise and the thought of going to the gym is making you want to take a nap, think of different ways to break your sedentary time and how you can increase your activity. Cycle to work or school instead of driving. If that is not possible, park further away from your office so you force yourself into two 15-minute walks every day. When you go shopping, park at the end of the car park instead of driving around for a spot near the door.
- Move more; walk your dog more often or clean your house more vigorously. If you own a Fitbit, Apple Watch or other fitness tracker, use it to check how many calories you can burn just by dusting, cleaning your bathroom, mowing the lawn, working in the garden, vacuuming and sweeping – all those tasks can give you a good workout. Studies have shown that breaking up sedentary time, even

if only for a couple of minutes can be beneficial to your health. Try exercising at your desk – it's totally possible to turn your office job into a calorie-burning activity. Standing desks are a good idea, and any office with stairs gives you an opportunity to break up your work routine.

● Have fun. What do you enjoy? What sounds like an activity you might like to try? You have lots of options, and again you don't have to go to a gym. Dancing, gardening, hiking, water aerobics or swimming are just a few ideas. Jenny belongs to a cycling club and teaches yoga. Giancarlo loves to work hard in the garden building a pond, moving earth or planting. Anything that raises your heart rate counts.

● Make moving a habit. Being fit means incorporating things into your life that eventually become a habit, just like starting your day with a cup of tea or coffee. To dispel the afternoon feeling of wanting a snack, do something else like walk around the office or the block to get some fresh air. Have a cup of tea when you return to your desk and you won't need the biscuit. After dinner, get into the habit of going out for a walk. Hunger pangs come and go, and often when you think you are hungry, you aren't, or the feeling will pass.

● Find someone to get fit with you. It is much more fun when you have an exercise buddy to share the pain and the gain. Create a plan which you can both commit to and keep each other on track. You could even get a group of people in on your "keep fit" mission to really motivate you.

● Buy a good pair of shoes. It's really important to own a good pair of trainers that are right for your chosen activity. As an example, jogging in tennis shoes is really not advised, as your foot needs a different type of support when you run. Dr Unwin ran in his brogues until he knew better!

● Hydrate. Drink water before, during and after exercise.

● Listen to your body. It is normal for your muscles to feel sore at first. However, you are unlikely to get injured unless you do too much too soon. Some of my clients get injured because they have the wrong, often competitive, attitude. It is far better to have a graduated approach and exercise safely.

The Next Step

Some of you will want to take getting fit more seriously, and high-intensity interval training is the most effective way to do this. However, anyone on medication should speak to their doctor first.

HIGH-INTENSITY INTERVAL TRAINING (HIIT)

HIIT is a faster route to fitness. Some people are naturally fit and can handle exertion well, while others systematically improve through repetition. In order to do HIIT successfully, you need to exert yourself to the point where you struggle to breathe and your muscles are screaming from burning. You then take a short break and do it again!

Many people will be petrified of this sort of workout, especially if they hate any form of exertion, so, if this is you, make sure you set yourself realistic goals and choose a workout you actually like doing. As you get fitter, you will become more resilient.

PARKRUN

Some GP surgeries have teamed up with parkrun.org.uk. These are local events where you turn up and walk, jog or run 5km. Check out their website for a run near you.

"It killed me at first, but now I look forward to the challenge and I can feel the effect and increased energy way after I have stopped exercising." Katie

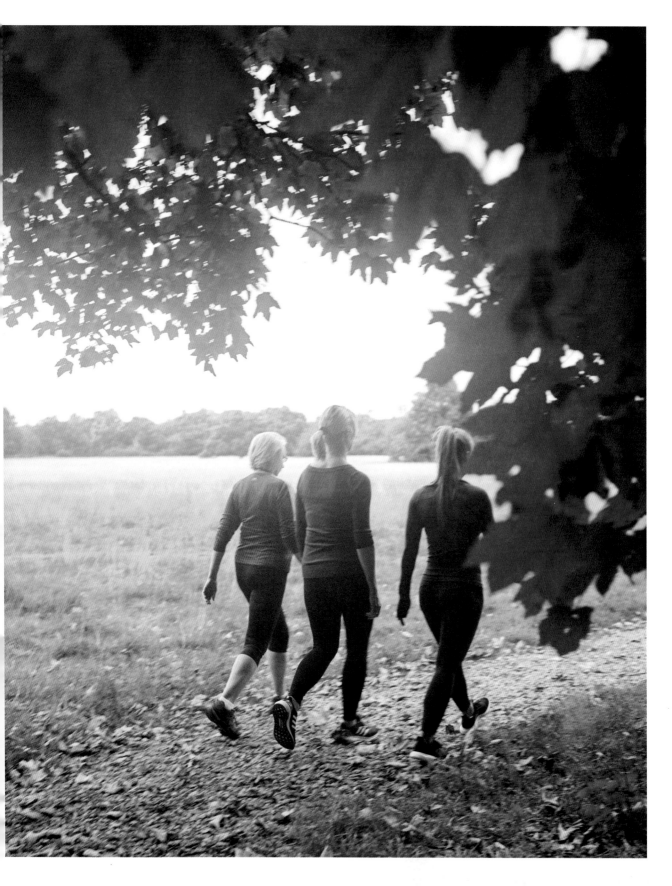

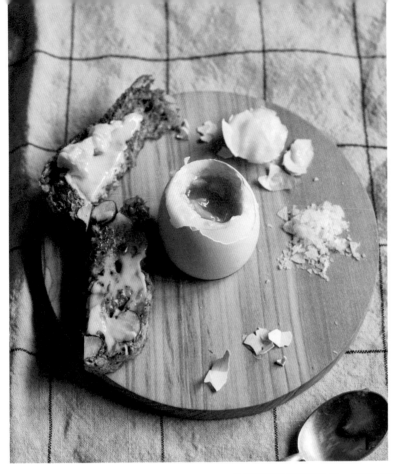

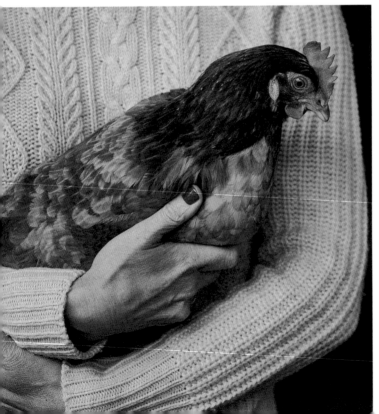

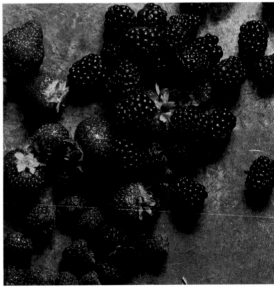

BREAKFAST *and* BRUNCH

Many people panic when they hear that cereal and toast are off the breakfast menu, but in fact now we often don't feel like food first thing in the morning – the hunger disappears when you follow a low-carb diet. Eating first thing is convention and the countless marketing ads telling us that breakfast is the most important meal of the day that get us in the habit. I used to be starving when I woke up, but I now frequently miss breakfast or opt for brunch instead.

When you do fancy breakfast, try to make sure you leave enough time to prepare something decent, rather than grabbing a sugary bun and latte on the way to work. You might be surprised and delighted to know that that when you are counting carbs it is much better to have a traditional English breakfast without the toast or a handful of walnuts and two squares of dark chocolate.

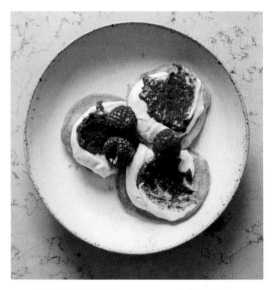

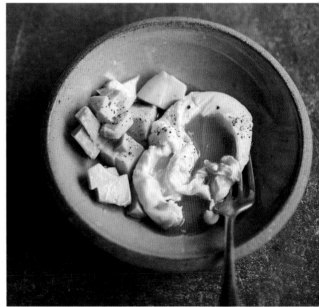

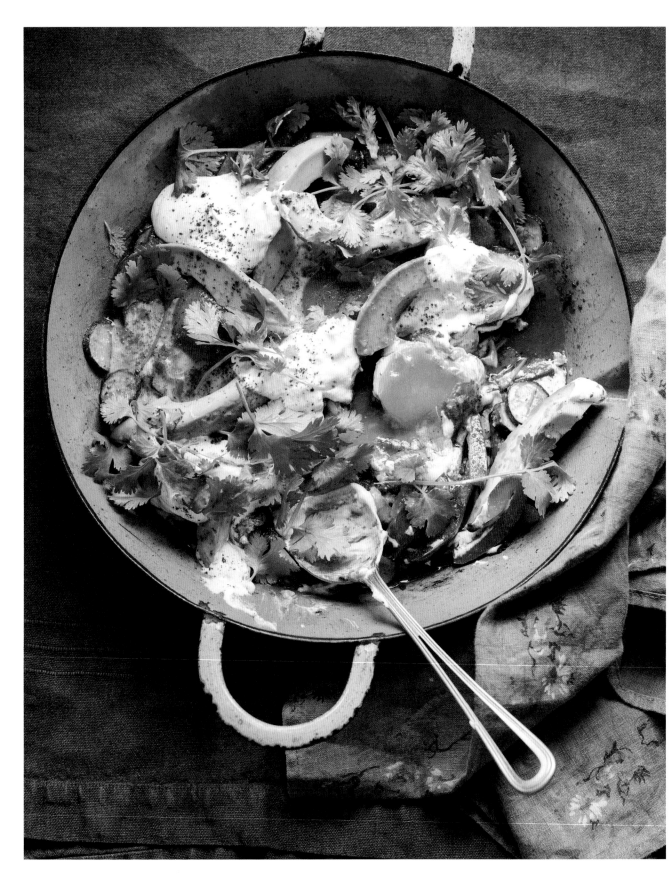

Turkish Eggs

Giancarlo says that when our friend Amal cooks she makes a picture with the food. It's true, particularly in her recipe for Turkish Eggs as it is so colourful and vibrant. Feel free to swap and change the vegetables; we often add sliced mushrooms or spring onions to the pan.

Heat the oil in a large, non-stick frying pan over a medium heat. Once hot, add the tomato sauce in a pool the centre of the pan. (If you are using canned tomatoes, season them.)

Lay the pepper and courgettes around the edge of the circle of sauce. Let the sauce heat up and the vegetables fry for 2 minutes, turning the pepper and courgettes as they brown. Season the vegetables in the pan. Don't be tempted to stir the sauce into the vegetables or they will boil and not fry.

Crack the eggs into the centre of the pan, over the sauce. Season the eggs, put the lid on the pan and leave to cook for 5 minutes, or until the eggs are done to your liking. Remove the lid and sprinkle over the cumin and turmeric. Lay the avocado around the edge, dollop on the yogurt and scatter the coriander over the top. Sprinkle with sumac and serve straight away on warm plates.

SERVES 2

2 tablespoons extra virgin olive oil
5 tablespoons Super Quick Tomato Sauce (page 90) or ½ x 400g (14oz) can of plum tomatoes, roughly chopped
1 red pepper, sliced into 1cm (½in) strips
2 baby courgettes or 1 small courgette, cut into 0.5cm (¼in) slices
4 eggs
¼ teaspoon ground cumin
¼ teaspoon ground turmeric
1 avocado, peeled, stoned and cut into 8 long wedges
5 heaped tablespoons Greek yogurt
a small handful of coriander leaves
salt and freshly ground black pepper
sumac, to serve

Per serving 12g carbs, 30g protein, 49g fat, 5.7g fibre, 631kcal

Poached Eggs in Tomato Sauce

This is Giancarlo's father's way to cook eggs, which in Italy is also known as 'Eggs in Purgatory' referring to the bubbling furnace of tomato sauce underneath. We keep a container of tomato sauce in the fridge so that we can whip these up for a quick breakfast or lunch. We serve them in a bowl with a spoon, but you could toast some low-carb bread (page 69) and pour the tomatoes on top.

Pour the tomato sauce into a wide frying pan and set over a medium heat. Break the eggs into the sauce, keeping them separate. Cover the pan with a lid and cook until the eggs have just cooked through – 5–7 minutes usually does it.

Scatter with basil, black pepper, Parmesan and a swirl of olive oil before serving.

SERVES 2

½ quantity Classic Tomato Sauce (page 90)
4 eggs
10 basil leaves
freshly ground black pepper
25g (1oz) finely grated Parmesan, to serve
extra virgin olive oil, to serve

Per serving: 10g carbs, 23g protein, 36g fat, 2.2g fibre, 466kcal

Giancarlo's Brunch

GIANCARLO'S MUSHROOMS

Giancarlo's way of cooking mushrooms is to "put the woods back into them" as he says. By adding herbs and garlic any mushroom tastes amazing.

Heat the oil in a large frying pan over a high heat. Add the garlic, thyme, rosemary and chilli, and season with a generous pinch of salt and pepper.

Fry for 1 minute, then add the mushrooms and cook them over a high heat, tossing or stirring frequently for 10–15 minutes. Allow the water to evaporate from the mushrooms as they cook; this will concentrate their flavour.

Eat straight away or cool and keep covered in the fridge for up to 4 days.

SERVES 4

3 tablespoons extra virgin olive oil
2 garlic cloves, lightly crushed
3 large sprigs of thyme
3–4 sprigs of rosemary
½–1 red chilli (according to taste), finely sliced
500g (18oz) chestnut, button or portobello mushrooms, brushed clean and thickly sliced
salt and freshly ground black pepper

Per 130g serving *4.6g carbs, 3.1g protein, 1.6g fat, 1.4g fibre, 47kcal*

OVEN-BAKED TOMATOES

These are just wonderful with grilled meats and fish or mozzarella and basil. Use any ripe, flavourful tomatoes to make this useful side dish.

Preheat the oven to 200°C/fan 180°C/gas mark 6.

Cut the tomatoes in half (around the equator, not pole to pole) and lay on a baking tray. Season with salt and pepper. Bake for 15 minutes. Remove the tray from the oven and scatter over the oregano and oil.

Return to the oven for 5–15 minutes or until the tomatoes just start to collapse and brown. Serve warm.

SERVES 4 as a starter, side or antipasti

400g (14oz) ripe flavourful tomatoes
1 teaspoon finely chopped oregano
3 tablespoons extra virgin olive oil
salt and freshly ground black pepper

Per 75g serving *3g carbs, 0.5g protein, 9.6g fat, 1g fibre, 106kcal*

DRY-FRIED HALLOUMI

Warm slices of halloumi are wonderful to eat, on their own, with a salad or soup. Eat them as soon as they are cooked, when they are still soft.

Cut the halloumi cheese into cubes or slices as you wish. Heat a non-stick frying pan over a medium-high heat. Add the cheese to the pan. Water sometimes comes out of the cheese – allow this to evaporate away.

Turn the cheese when it is lightly browned all over. Eat straight away or the cheese becomes firm and squeaky again quite quickly.

SERVES 4

250g (9oz) halloumi cheese

Per 60g serving *1g carbs, 15g protein, 15g fat, 0.7g fibre, 196kcal*

TO SERVE
Divide the halloumi, tomatoes and mushrooms between four plates. Add avocado for a substantial vegetarian brunch.

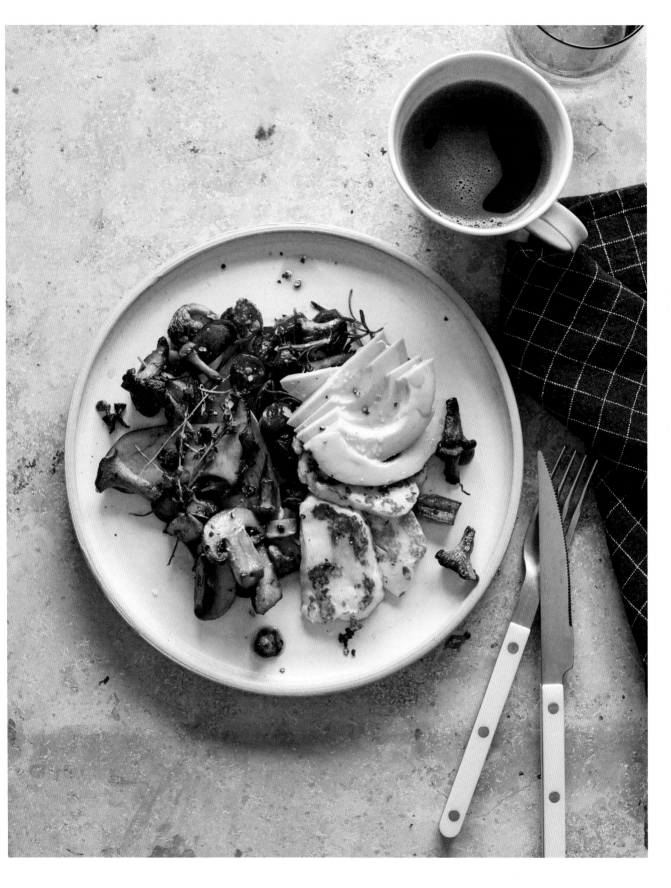

Mushrooms with Spinach, Poached Eggs & Cheat's Hollandaise Sauce

This version of hollandaise sauce is so easy to make; keep the heat low, don't leave the pan and you will have perfect results every time. We love it poured over freshly steamed asparagus, too.

We have prepared the spinach in the microwave as we find it the easiest method, but by all means use sautéed fresh spinach leaves instead. If you are feeling hungry, cook two eggs each or add a thick slice of smoked ham under the eggs.

Preheat the grill to hot.

Lay the mushrooms, cut-side up, on a wire rack over a baking tray, brush with the oil and season.

Grill for 7–10 minutes or until tender and darker around the edges. Using tongs, turn the mushrooms over so the bottoms are upwards and grill for 3–5 minutes. Remove from the grill when cooked through and set aside. Bring a large frying pan of water to the boil for the eggs.

To make the sauce, put all the ingredients into a small saucepan over a gentle heat and warm through until the butter has melted. Keep stirring for a minute or two and remove from the heat. Season to taste.

To poach the eggs, reduce the heat and let the water simmer gently. Crack one of the eggs into a teacup and partially submerge the cup in the water. Let the egg slide out into the water disturbing it as little as possible. Do the same with the remaining eggs. Allow 3 minutes for soft-boiled and lift them out one at a time with a slotted spoon. Set aside on a warm plate until you are ready to serve.

When the mushrooms are cooked, put them on warm plates, top with the warm spinach followed by a poached egg. Pour over the sauce and add a twist of pepper to each one. Serve straight away.

SERVES 4

4 large portobello mushrooms, brushed clean and stalks cut away
1 tablespoon extra virgin olive oil
4 eggs
salt and freshly ground black pepper
1 quantity Cheat's Creamy Spinach (page 178), or 200g (7oz) cooked and squeezed spinach, to serve

For the sauce
3 tablespoons homemade or shop-bought mayonnaise
½ teaspoon Dijon mustard
2 teaspoons lemon juice
2 tablespoons double cream
4 tablespoons salted butter

Per serving *3.7g carbs, 15g protein, 63g fat, 5.7g fibre, 653kcal*

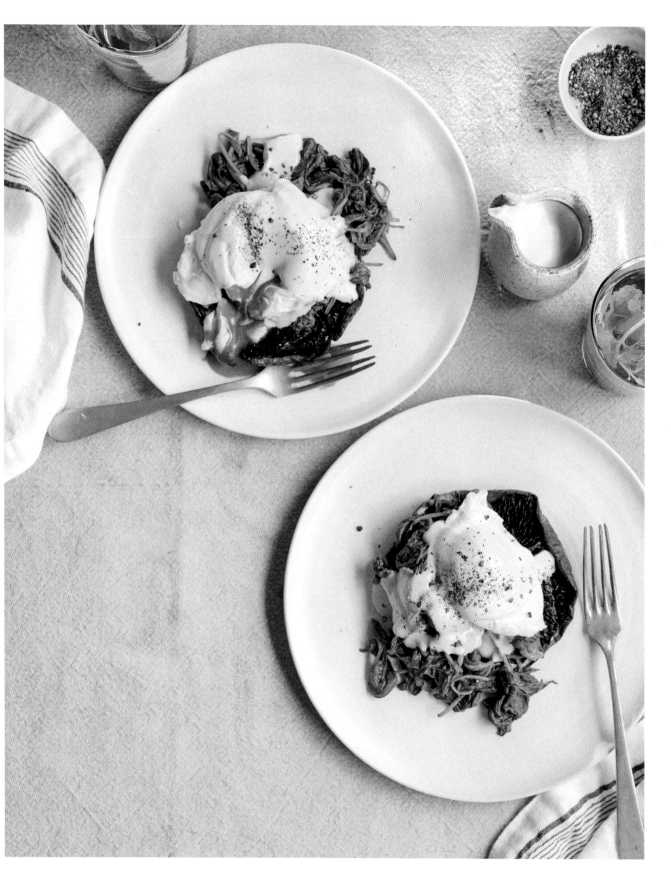

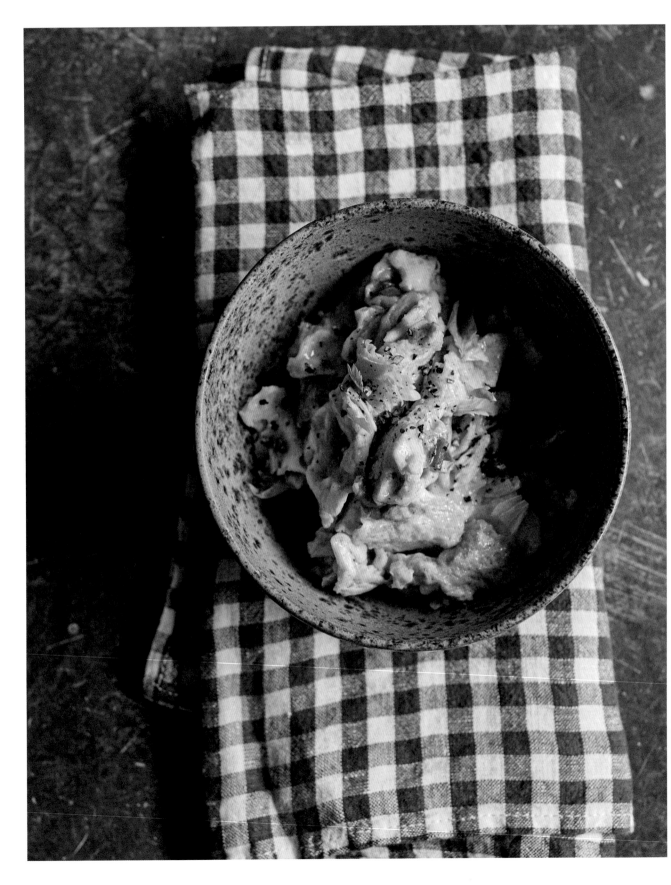

Scrambled Eggs with Celery Leaves

Celery leaves, so often discarded, add a spice to eggs. They are surprisingly tasty and a breakfast like this only takes a couple of minutes. Serve it on its own, or with smoked salmon or spoonfuls of goat's cheese, and if you don't have celery leaves, use parsley, chives or fresh oregano instead.

Whisk the eggs with the celery leaves and seasoning in a bowl while you warm a non-stick frying pan over a medium heat. Add the butter and, when it has just started to bubble and spread, pour the egg mixture into the centre.

When the edges have just started to set, use a silicone spatula to gently stir the eggs to create waves. Keep folding and moving the eggs around for 2 minutes until the eggs are just set.

Remove from the heat and serve on warm plates with the tomatoes. Dress with a swirl of olive oil, another twist of pepper and a little salt on the tomatoes.

SERVES 2

4 eggs
2 tablespoons coarsely chopped
 celery leaves
knob of butter or ghee, or
 2 tablespoons extra virgin olive oil
salt and freshly ground black pepper
6 cherry tomatoes, halved, to serve
extra virgin olive oil, to serve

Per serving *2g carbs, 16g protein, 13g fat, 0.7g fibre, 195kcal*

Courgette, Broccoli & Halloumi Scramble

I can make this dish in roughly 12 minutes and eat it regularly for breakfast. We add more eggs and halloumi for our teenage boys and they love it for lunch or supper. It's a great way to use up leftover vegetables, herbs, spinach leaves or cooked meat; toss them into the pan and heat through before adding the eggs.

Heat the oil in a large, non-stick frying pan and add the courgette, broccoli, spring onions, chilli and seasoning (go easy with the salt as the halloumi can be salty). Add 3 tablespoons of water. Put the lid on and cook, shaking the pan frequently, for 7–10 minutes until the vegetables are just tender.

Meanwhile, dry-fry the cubes of halloumi in a non-stick frying pan (see page 54).

Remove the lid from the pan with the vegetables and allow the water to evaporate if there is any left. Add the eggs, halloumi and parsley. Stir with a spatula until the egg is just cooked through and serve straight away.

SERVES 2

2 tablespoons extra virgin olive oil,
 ghee or butter
1 courgette, cut into 1cm (½in) circles
100g (3½oz) broccoli, cut into small
 florets
3 spring onions, roughly chopped
a few slices of green or red chilli or
 pinch of chilli flakes
125g (4½oz) halloumi, cut into dice
4 eggs, beaten
a handful of parsley, roughly chopped
salt and freshly ground black pepper

Per serving *4g carbs, 32g protein, 27g fat, 3.3g fibre, 390kcal*

Smoked Salmon & Dill Breakfast Eggs

This lovely breakfast takes just the right amount of time to cook while you have a shower and get dressed. Alternatively, it makes a good light lunch if served with a salad on the side. The mixture rises like a soufflé and can be eaten from the hot ramekin or turned out onto a plate. If you don't eat fish, stir in some cooked spinach or buttered leeks instead. Offcuts of smoked salmon are ideal for this recipe.

Preheat the oven to 220°C/fan 200°C/gas mark 7. Generously butter a ramekin dish to allow the mixture to rise easily and turn out if you wish.

Beat the egg with the crème fraîche and a small pinch of salt and pepper. Now stir in the salmon and dill. Pour the mixture into the buttered ramekin dish. Put onto a baking tray and bake for 15–20 minutes, or until just set. Leave to cool for a couple of minutes before serving.

SERVES 1

butter, for greasing
1 egg
1 heaped tablespoon crème fraîche or double cream
50g (2oz) smoked salmon flakes or smoked salmon, roughly cut
few sprigs of dill, roughly chopped
salt and freshly ground black pepper

Per 177g serving 1.5g carbs, 21g protein, 38g fat, 0g fibre, 436kcal

Cinnamon Granola

Instead of the sugar-laden granola you can buy in the shops, try this easy way to make your own. We have added two dates for just a hint of sweetness, but if you are on the lower end of the CarbScale leave them out. Do store the granola out of sight; if I leave it out at home it gets eaten within a day – it's so moreish!
   Turmeric is a powerful anti-inflammatory and the black pepper and the fat in the nuts help it to be absorbed by your body. We use almonds, pecans and pistachios for the nuts and a mixture of pumpkin, sunflower and sesame seeds.

Preheat the oven to 200°C/fan 180°C/gas mark 6. Line a baking tray with a silicone baking mat or baking parchment.

Put the dates into a large mixing bowl and add the boiling water. Use a fork to mash them to a thick pulp. Add the remaining ingredients and mix thoroughly. Spread the mixture onto the lined baking tray and bake for 10–12 minutes until lightly browned. Remove from the oven and set aside to cool. Store in an airtight container for up to 2 weeks.

MAKES APPROX. 450G (1LB)/ SERVES 18 (25G/1OZ PORTIONS)

2 Medjool dates, stoned and finely chopped
2 tablespoons boiling water
300g (10½oz) mixed nuts
60g (2½oz) mixed seeds
2 tablespoons flaxseeds (optional)
25g (1oz) desiccated coconut
2 teaspoons vanilla extract
50g (2oz) unsalted butter or coconut oil
2 teaspoons ground cinnamon
1 teaspoon ground turmeric (optional)
½ teaspoon freshly ground black pepper (optional)

Per 25g serving 2.7g carbs, 3.9g protein, 15g fat, 2.2g fibre, 166kcal

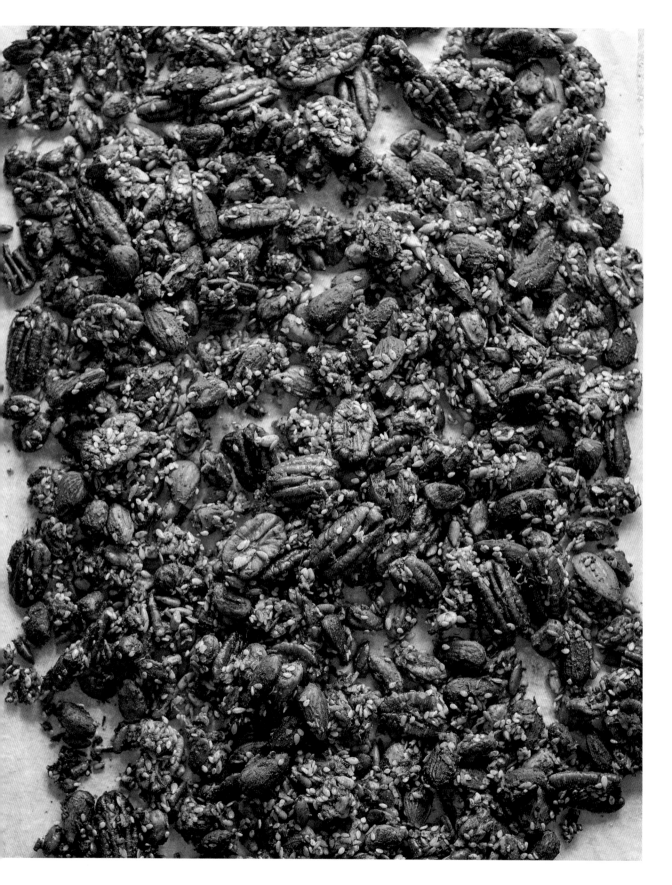

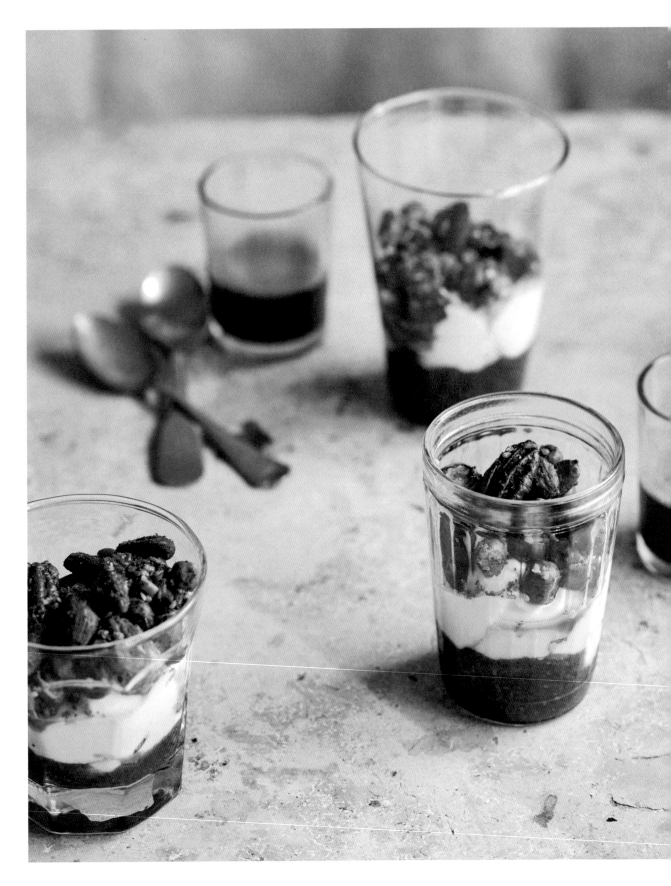

Greek Yogurt with Blueberries, Cinnamon Granola & Raspberry Jam

This recipe is so easy to whip up and is great for a healthy breakfast or a pudding. We like to use small glasses to show off the colourful layers. The tiny little white or black seeds from the chia plant have a magical way of thickening sauces without the added carbs. If you use white chia seeds they will keep the jam bright red, but black chia work the same magic. By blending the seeds with the fruit they break up and work instantly. The jam will keep for four days chilled. If you prefer, use two ripe peaches or nectarines, stoned and cubed, instead of the blueberries. If you have it, add a drizzle of Vanilla Oil on top.

To make the **vanilla oil**, simply put the oil in a jar and mix with the seeds of the vanilla pod and the bean cut into a few pieces. Screw on the lid and leave in a cool, dark place for at least 3 days for the flavour to develop. Shake the jar before using and drizzle sparingly. We make small amounts of this to use on yogurt or fruit in place of honey.

To make the **raspberry chia jam**, whizz the raspberries with the chia seeds in a food-processor for 2 minutes or until the seeds have broken up.

Taste the mixture and, if the raspberries are sour, add some vanilla to taste. If the berries are still not sweet enough, dissolve the date in 3 tablespoons of boiling water by mashing it with a fork. Add it to the food-processor. Whizz again to combine. (If you don't have a food-processor, mix the ingredients by hand and wait an hour; the mixture will thicken up all the same.)

Put 1 tablespoon of jam in the bottom of each small glass and top with 3 tablespoons of yogurt. Follow with the blueberries, then another layer of jam and yogurt. (Or you can put all the jam at the bottom of each jar and top with the yogurt, if you wish.) Top each one with the cinnamon granola and/or a few whole blueberries. Eat straight away or store for up to a day in the fridge.

SERVES 6

500g (18oz) natural, thick, full-fat cow's, goat's or coconut milk yogurt
200g (7oz) blueberries
150g (5oz) Cinnamon Granola (page 60), or 60g (2½oz) mixed seeds or walnuts, roughly chopped

For the vanilla oil
100ml extra virgin olive oil
1 vanilla pod

For the Raspberry Chia Jam
300g (10½oz) raspberries, strawberries or blueberries, or a mixture
2 tablespoons chia seeds (milled or whole)
1 teaspoon vanilla extract or ½ teaspoon vanilla powder, to taste
1 Medjool date, stoned (optional)

Per serving 15g carbs, 10g protein, 24g fat, 7.4g fibre, 330kcal
Per serving of Raspberry Chia Jam 2.6g carbs, 1.3g protein, 1.2g fat, 4.6g fibre, 42kcal

Coconut Pancakes, Whipped Coconut Cream & Raspberries

There is no sugar in these pancakes, but they are naturally sweet from the coconut and vanilla, so they make a guilt-free breakfast, brunch or dessert. Coconut flour is made from the dried flesh of the coconut. It is high in fibre and works as a binder. It is also very absorbent, so you can't simply swap it for wheat flour as it needs much more liquid. These pancakes are delicious served with Raspberry Chia Jam (page 63), or simply with a few berries. The coconut cream is also gorgeous on desserts, or stirred into coffee. Make sure you have a 400ml (14fl oz) can of coconut milk that has been left in the fridge or a cool cupboard before you start, so it has time to separate into the denser cream at the top and the water below; don't shake it.

To make the whipped coconut cream, carefully spoon the cream out of the can leaving the water below for the pancakes.

Whisk it in a bowl with the vanilla for a couple of minutes until thick and firm. Leave in a cool place until you are ready to serve.

Whisk the eggs with the vanilla and coconut water or milk in a large bowl. In another bowl, mix the dry ingredients.

Little by little add the dry ingredients to the wet, whisking all the time until you have a thick cream consistency.

Heat a large, non-stick frying pan over a medium heat and add the fat. When melted and just starting to bubble, swirl the fat around the pan to coat it. Drop 1 tablespoon measures of the batter into the pan, making sure they don't touch as they spread out. Use a fish slice or spatula to gently turn the pancakes when they are set and firm on one side. They will take 3–4 minutes on the first side and only 1–2 minutes on the second.

Remove the pancakes from the pan when done and serve straight away or keep warm while you make the rest. Serve with the whipped coconut cream and raspberry chia jam and some raspberries, if you wish.

MAKES APPROX. 16 PANCAKES (ABOUT 6CM/2½IN ACROSS)/ SERVES 6

4 eggs
1 teaspoon vanilla extract or ½ teaspoon vanilla powder
120ml (4fl oz) coconut water from the can, coconut milk or cow's milk
1 teaspoon baking powder
4 tablespoons coconut flour
small pinch of salt
2 tablespoons coconut oil, ghee or butter, for frying

For the whipped coconut cream
approx. 130g (4½oz) coconut cream (from the top of the can or bought separately), chilled
1 teaspoon vanilla extract or ½ teaspoon vanilla powder

Per pancake: 1.1g carbs, 0.6g protein, 3.1g fat, 0.9g fibre, 37kcal
Per serving of whipped cream 1.2g carbs, 0.9g protein, 6.9g fat, 0g fibre, 74kcal

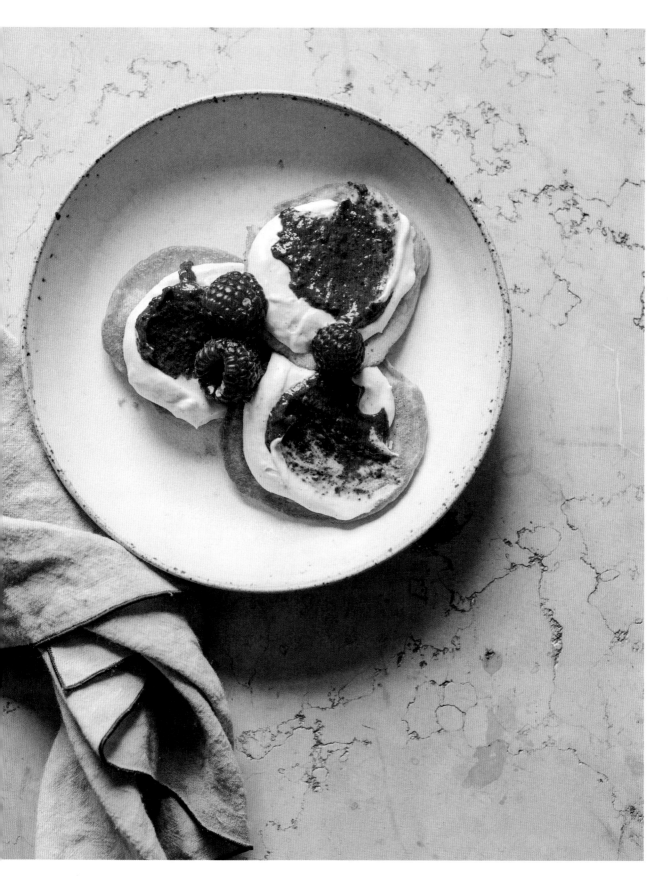

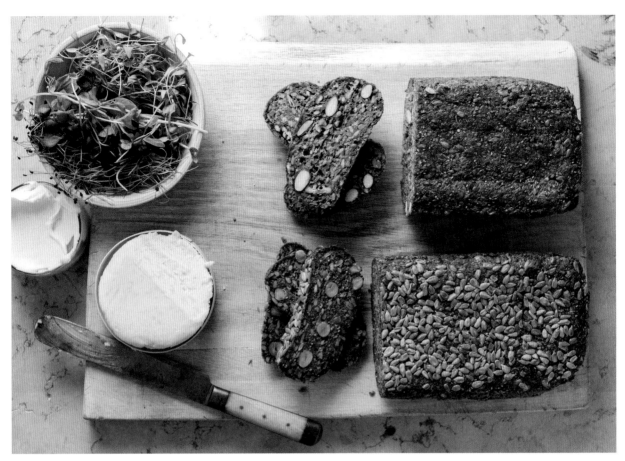

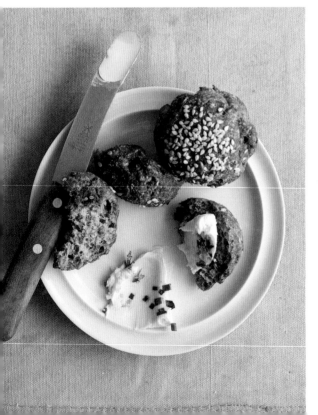

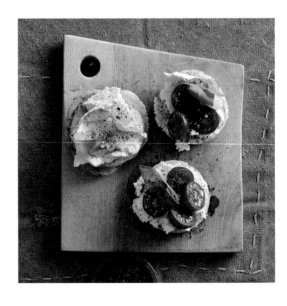

BREADS, PIZZA, CRACKERS and PASTRY

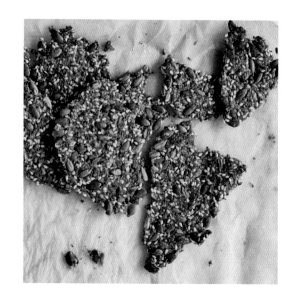

One of the hardest foods to give up when you go low-carb is bread. As a keen breadmaker I was determined not to substitute my homemade wheat bread with anything inferior. After years of experimenting with gluten-free and low-carb, we are really happy with the recipes in this chapter. They are every bit as good as traditional breads, and now Giancarlo and the family can enjoy pizza, muffins, focaccia and wraps once again.

We keep our bread in small bags in the freezer, each holding two slices, ready to toast or defrost for a sandwich. That way you are less likely to go on eating your way through a loaf when you see it in the bread bin. The pizza base freezes well, too, and takes minutes to thaw.

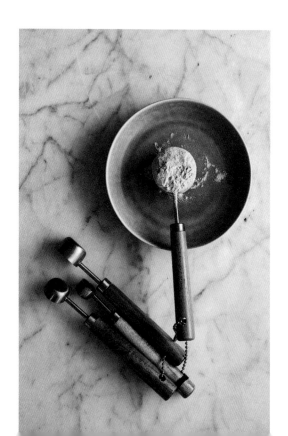

Scandi Seeded Crackers with Avocado & Yogurt Dip

We ate these seed-speckled crackers in Sweden with lashings of butter. This recipe is from our Finnish friend Lorna Smalley; they are not only incredibly moreish but low-carb, wheat-free and highly nutritious.

The crackers are served broken up into shards (see photo on page 67). They are delicious with mashed avocado, cheese or smoked salmon. Try flavouring the crackers with dried herbs or seeds such as onion seeds, cumin or caraway. They keep well in an airtight container for up to a week. The dip is also a great dressing for salmon, chicken, salad or boiled eggs.

Preheat the oven to 200°C/fan 180°C/gas mark 6. Line a baking tray with baking parchment and lightly brush it with oil.

Thoroughly mix the ingredients together in a large mixing bowl, adding 5–6 tablespoons of cold water to form a thick paste. Use a spatula to scrape the mixture onto the lined tray.

Take another piece of baking parchment the size of your baking tray and brush it with oil. Put this, oil side down, on top of the mixture and roll it with a short rolling pin or an empty wine bottle so that the cracker mixture is about 2mm (¹/₁₆in) thick.

Remove the top piece of parchment and put the tray into the oven to cook for 18–20 minutes, or until lightly browned and brittle.

Meanwhile, blend the ingredients for the dip together in a bowl with a fork or in a food-processor and adjust the taste accordingly. It will keep for up to 3 days in the fridge in a covered bowl or Kilner jar.

Once cool enough to touch, break the baked cracker mixture into shards. If any of the crackers look undercooked underneath, simply put them back in the oven for a couple of minutes to crisp up. Once they are bone dry, they will keep in an airtight container for a week.

SERVES 8

extra virgin olive oil, to grease
150g (5oz) mixed seeds, such as sunflower, pumpkin, poppy, hemp, coriander, sesame, black onion, cumin, caraway
50g (2oz) milled flaxseed
1 tablespoon psyllium husk powder
½ teaspoon fine salt
1 egg white (30g/1¼oz)
1 teaspoon dried oregano (optional)

For the avocado and yogurt dip
150ml (5fl oz) full-fat Greek yogurt
2 avocados, peeled, stoned and roughly chopped
juice of 1 small lemon
1 garlic clove, finely grated
salt and freshly ground black pepper

Per 30g (1oz) serving of crackers *3.1g carbs, 6g protein, 11g fat, 3.9g fibre, 147kcal*

Per serving of dip *1.5g carbs, 2.5g protein, 8.1g fat, 1.2g fibre, 92kcal*

Low-carb Bread

This bread brings a smile to Giancarlo's face every time I make it. Finally he gets the joy of tearing and eating bread without the gluten and carbs. I love to alter the texture with the addition of seeds and nuts, and the recipe adapts well to various shapes. The bread, once cooked and cooled, lasts for 3 days in the bread bin and it freezes well too.

One word of warning, the psyllium husk firms up as it cools, so no nibbling on the bread before it is at room temperature or you will find a soggy dough consistency. Our recipe is an adaptation of one from Maria Emmerich and her inspiring website: mariamindbodyhealth.com. Add leftover egg yolks to scrambled eggs in the morning.

Preheat the oven to 200°C/fan 180°C/gas mark 6. Grease a baking tray with a little oil.

Mix the dry ingredients in the bowl of a stand mixer or food-processor.

Pour the water into the dry mixture and stir through with a dough hook or plastic blade. (You can do this by hand with a metal spoon, but mixers are easier.) Add the eggs and mix once more to combine.

Remove the dough from the bowl and drizzle a little oil onto your hands. It is now ready to shape into the following variations.

To make baguettes, roll and stretch the dough into two even-sized long baguettes with lightly oiled hands. Each one will be about 35cm (14in) long – just shorter than the length of a baking tray – and about 6cm (2½in) wide.

Lay them onto the greased tray and sprinkle with seeds (if using). Bake for 50 minutes or until they sound hollow. Leave to cool to room temperature before cutting and eating.

MAKES 1 FOCACCIA OR 2 BAGUETTES/SERVES 8 OR 20 MINI-ROLLS/SERVES 10

extra virgin olive oil, to grease the tray and shape the dough
150g (5oz) almond flour or ground almonds
5 tablespoons ground psyllium husk powder
2 teaspoons baking powder
½ teaspoon fine sea salt
250ml (9fl oz) boiling water
3 medium eggs
2 tablespoons seeds, to decorate (optional)

Per serving 2.3g carbs, 8.1g protein, 14g fat, 12g fibre, 194kcal

Variations to add to the dough

- 100g (3½oz) finely chopped mixed herbs, such as basil, parsley, celery leaves, oregano or chives
- 6 tablespoons seeds, such as sesame, sunflower, poppy or pumpkin
- 50g (2oz) finely grated Parmesan or other hard cheese and 2 handfuls of chopped chives
- 100g (3½oz) finely chopped sun-dried tomatoes and 2 tablespoons finely chopped rosemary leaves
- 2 large handfuls of chopped olives and 2 tablespoons fennel seeds
- 4 teaspoons caraway seeds for a Swedish flavour to go on the Smörgåsbord on page 128

Walnut & Parmesan Seeded Rolls with Herb Butter

These small bread rolls are perfect for entertaining when served warm with Herb Butter (see below) or they are great for taking to work with a filling of your choice. The recipe can be added to with sun-dried tomatoes, chopped nuts or other flavourings as you wish, see the list below. The cheese can be omitted, too – it's fun to experiment. The rolls will last for about 3 days in a cool place in a paper bag. If your house is warm, keep them in the fridge and warm up in the oven before using.

Preheat the oven to 200°C/fan 180°C/gas mark 6.

Add the walnuts, cheese, seeds and some black pepper into the bowl with the dough and use your hands to combine them together. Drizzle a little oil onto your hands and shape the dough into even-sized rolls about 4cm (1½in) across.

Lay the rolls spaced apart by at least 6cm (2½in) onto a baking tray. Flatten the rolls down a little and at this point press in a few extra seeds, if you like.

Bake for 35–40 minutes, or until the rolls sound hollow when tapped and are firm to the touch. Remove from the oven and leave to cool to room temperature on a wire rack before serving.

MAKES 20 MINI ROLLS (ABOUT 6CM/2½IN ACROSS)/SERVES 10

50g (2oz) roughly chopped walnuts
25g (1oz) Parmesan, finely grated
3 heaped tablespoons seeds (sunflower, pumpkin, sesame), plus extra (optional) to decorate
1 quantity Low-carb Bread dough (page 69)
extra virgin olive oil, to shape the dough
freshly ground black pepper

Per serving with butter
2.8g carbs, 9.2g protein, 22g fat, 9.8g fibre, 269kcal

Herb butter

Mould a 250g (9oz) block of salted or unsalted butter into a thick circle on a small wooden board or serving plate. Now let your imagination run riot! Arrange rows of finely chopped fresh herbs, such as chives, oregano, thyme, chive flowers or mint, on top. Alternate the herbs with salt flakes, lemon zest or finely chopped red chilli. Serve.

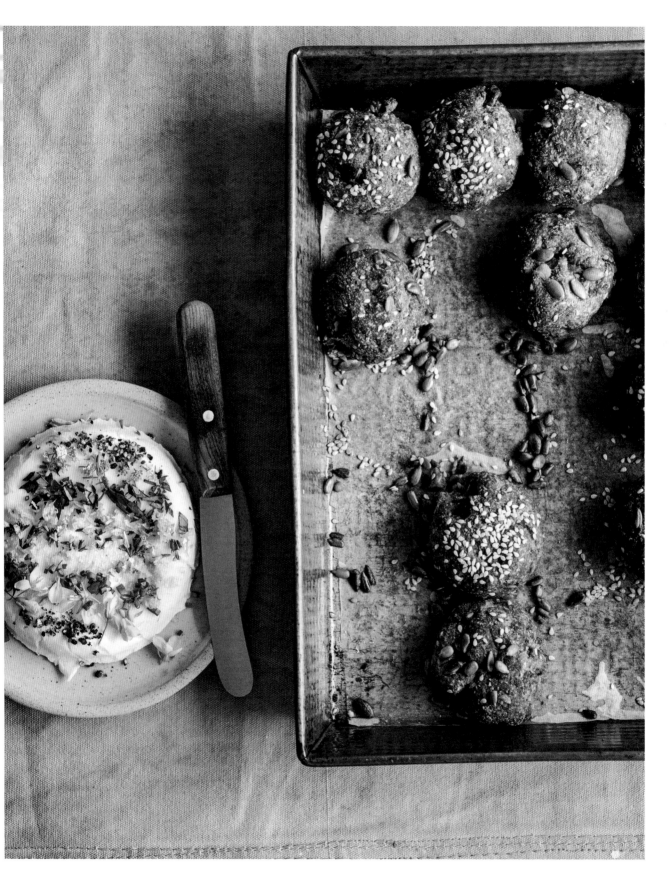

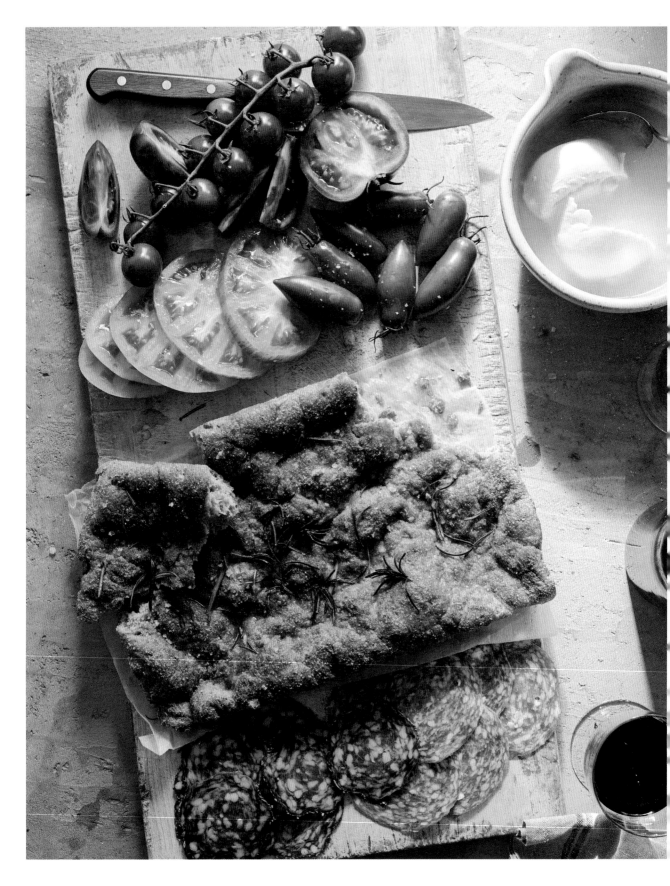

Rosemary Focaccia

When pushed for time, paired with delicious antipasti, this is my go-to starter or meal when friends or family descend. You can bake a low-carb Rosemary Focaccia in 30 minutes and at the same time rustle up some Rosemary-roasted Pecans (page 45).

Preheat the oven to 200°C/fan 180°C/gas mark 6.

Spread the dough out onto a sheet of baking parchment or a silicone mat to 1cm (½in) thick – it will be about 20cm (8in) in length and 17cm (6½in) wide. Make indentations in the surface with your fingers.

Drizzle over the oil and scatter over a good pinch of salt flakes. Tuck in small sprigs of rosemary leaves and bake for 30 minutes or until browned and cooked through.

Remove from the oven and leave to cool and for the psyllium husk to settle and set. When you are ready to serve, put the focaccia back in the oven for 5 minutes to warm and serve drizzled with a little oil.

SERVES 4

1 quantity Low-carb Bread dough recipe (page 69)
2 tablespoons extra virgin olive oil, plus extra to finish
salt flakes
2 sprigs of rosemary

Per serving *2.3g carbs, 8.1g protein, 14g fat, 12g fibre, 194kcal*

Italian antipasti

Stock up on prosciutto, buffalo mozzarella, tomatoes, basil and a good olive oil. Get out your biggest wooden chopping board and get arranging. Mozzarella should be torn and sat on top of sliced tomatoes with basil leaves, pepper and salt and a good drizzle of extra virgin olive oil. Prosciutto works like a flavour enhancer – try it wrapped around basil leaves and bocconcini (baby mozzarella), or rolled around the humble celery stick. Lay out some olives, cubes of cheese and salami and serve the focaccia warm.

Seed & Nut Loaf

This dense nutty brown loaf is adapted from Sarah Britton's Life-Changing Loaf recipe that she developed while living in Denmark. The bread did literally change her life as the recipe from her blog – www.mynewroots.org – went viral. This is our version minus the maple syrup. You can use oats if you can't find quinoa flakes, but the carb count is higher.

This loaf is just gorgeous with butter, Marmite, cheese or pâté. As it is packed with nuts and seeds it has a high fat content, so don't scoff too much in one go.

Put the dry ingredients into a large mixing bowl and stir to combine. Add 475ml (17floz) of cold water and stir through with a metal spoon to form a firm, heavy dough. Leave to firm up for 15 minutes.

Preheat the oven to 200°C/fan 180°C/gas mark 6. Line the base and long sides of a loaf tin with a long rectangle of baking parchment that flaps over the sides to help lift the loaf out. Grease the short ends. Alternatively, use a silicone loaf mould.

Use your hands to transfer the dough into the tin and flatten down the top, scattering over the extra sunflower seeds (if using). Bake for 45 minutes. Slide a knife around the loaf and tip it out of the tin using the paper. Put it onto a rack in the oven and remove the paper. Bake it for a further 30 minutes until it sounds hollow when tapped and is firm to the touch.

Remove the loaf from the oven and leave to cool to room temperature on a wire rack before slicing. If not freezing, store in a bag or sealed container for up to 5 days in the fridge or a cool place.

MAKES 1 LOAF
(16 finger-width slices)

135g (4¾oz) sunflower seeds, plus
  1 tablespoon extra (optional)
  to finish
60g (2½oz) ground flaxseeds
65g (2½oz) hazelnuts or almonds
75g (2¾oz) quinoa flakes or oats
2 tablespoons chia seeds, ground
3 tablespoons psyllium husk powder
1 teaspoon fine salt
oil, to grease

Per slice 5.1g carbs, 4.5g protein, 9.1g fat, 5.7g fibre, 131kcal

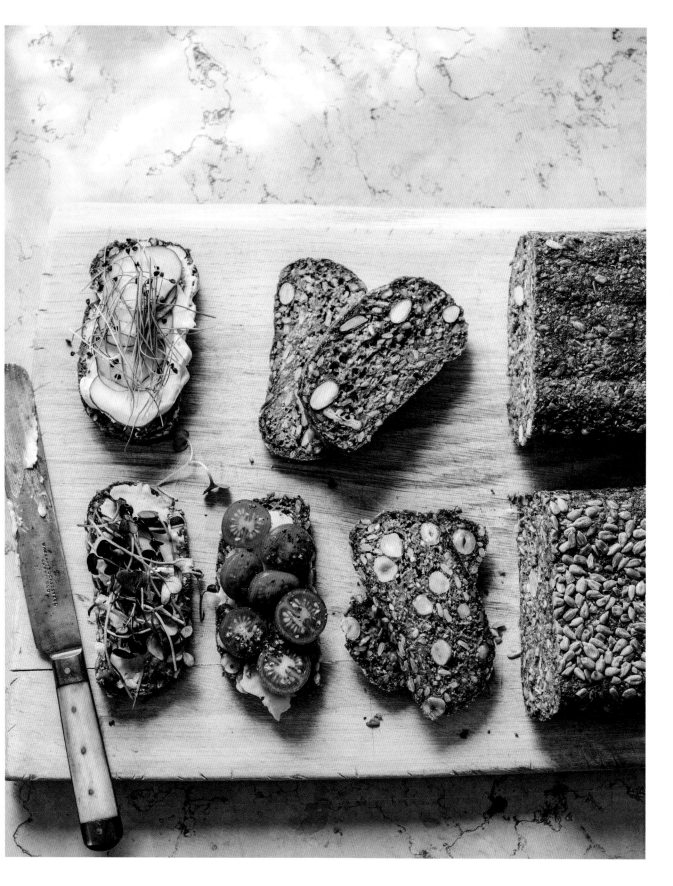

Flammekueche

This old recipe from Alsace is a type of flatbread topped with a mixture of cream, soft white cheese, bacon and onions. It was traditionally baked on the dying heat from the oven floor after the baker had finished cooking loaves, hence the name meaning "flame cake". Do also try topping them with cream cheese and Cinnamon & Brandy Buttered Apples (page 192).

Preheat the oven to 240°C/fan 220°C/gas mark 9 or as hot as your oven will go.

Heat the fat in a frying pan, add the shallot or onion and cook for 5 minutes, or until soft. Add the bacon and cook until just opaque.

In a mixing bowl, beat the cream cheese and crème fraîche together with the mustard, and season to taste.

Put the wraps onto a large baking tray and top with the cream mixture followed by the shallot and bacon. Swirl the oil over the top and bake for 5–7 minutes or until browned and crisp around the edges. Serve hot.

MAKES 2 FLAMMEKUECHE

1 tablespoon butter, ghee or extra virgin olive oil
1 shallot or ½ red or white onion, finely sliced into half moons
50g (2oz) lardons or 2 rashers streaky smoked bacon, finely sliced
30g (1oz) cream cheese
30g (1oz) crème fraîche
1 teaspoon Dijon mustard
2 Wraps (page 81)
1 tablespoon extra virgin olive oil
salt and freshly ground black pepper

Per flammekeuche 11g carbs, 13g protein, 33g fat, 5g fibre, 400kcal.

Psyllium husk powder

Psyllium husk powder or ground psyllium is the husk from the *plantago ovata* plant grown mainly in India. The husk is high in fibre so it is often used as a laxative. It becomes a gel when mixed with water and works like gluten as a binder. It can turn your baking a rich purpley-brown, but if you prefer golden-coloured bread look for blonde psyllium instead. If you buy "husk" rather than "husk powder" grind it to a powder in a food-processor before using. Keep blitzing it until it is half its original volume and use in recipes as husk powder. Psyllium is available online and in Asian and health food shops but avoid the expensive medicinal variety as the standard one will do.

Magic Muffins

This is an adaptation of the popular mug cake, but with a fraction of the carbs. This recipe comes from Katy Threlfall from Dr Unwin's low-carb patient group. As a busy mum, she makes one each day for a late breakfast or to carry with her when she is on the go.

The muffins can be eaten just as they are or topped with crème fraîche and strawberries. Alternatively, flavour the muffin mix with a pinch of ground cinnamon and top with almond butter and apple slices (see some ideas overleaf). If you make the mixture in a square container it can be sliced in two to make a sandwich. If you don't have a microwave, the muffins can be cooked in the oven for 10–15 minutes at 200°C/fan 180°C/ gas mark 6 but grease and line the container first.

Mix the egg and fat together. Add the ground almonds, baking powder, vanilla extract and fruit and mix well. Spoon into a small microwaveable pot or mug and microwave on full power for 3 minutes.

To make a **low-carb chocolate ganache** for the muffins or to eat on its own with raspberries (page 183), briefly melt equal measures of dark chocolate and cream together either in the microwave or in a bowl over a pan of simmering water and stir to combine.

MAKES I STANDARD-SIZED MUG MUFFIN

I egg
knob of butter, melted, or 2 teaspoons
  coconut oil or extra virgin olive oil
50g (2oz) ground almonds
½ teaspoon baking powder
½ teaspoon vanilla extract
½ apple or pear, grated

Per muffin 15g carbs, 21g protein, 42g fat, 7.5g fibre, 536kcal

Variations

FOR A SAVOURY MUFFIN
Use the standard recipe with ½ grated courgette, a good pinch of dried oregano, 15g (½oz) grated Parmesan and I tablespoon finely chopped coriander or parsley. After cooking the muffin, cut it into four slices and top with ricotta or cream cheese, cherry tomatoes, some torn basil leaves and black pepper.

FOR A CHOCOLATE VERSION
Use the pear or apple to sweeten the mixture and add I heaped teaspoon cocoa powder, ½ teaspoon vanilla extract and little shards of good-quality dark chocolate (85 per cent cocoa solids).

FOR MINI MUFFIN CANAPÉS
I made 60 of these and flavoured them with Arabic-inspired seasoning to serve at our Royal Wedding party.

The standard recipe for I mug muffin will make 12 mini muffins. Add I teaspoon ground cumin, I teaspoon black onion seeds, 2 tablespoons finely chopped coriander to the uncooked mixture. Spoon into a silicone mini muffin mould and bake at 200°C/fan 180°C/gas mark 6 for 12 minutes. Serve with a paste made of equal parts tahini and cream cheese. Balance ½ cherry tomato on top of each and add a little more coriander.

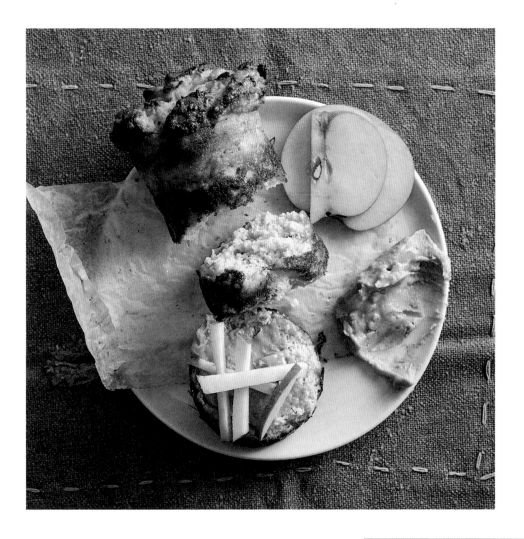

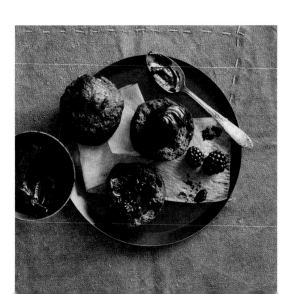

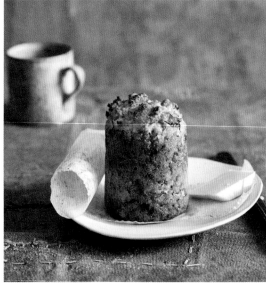

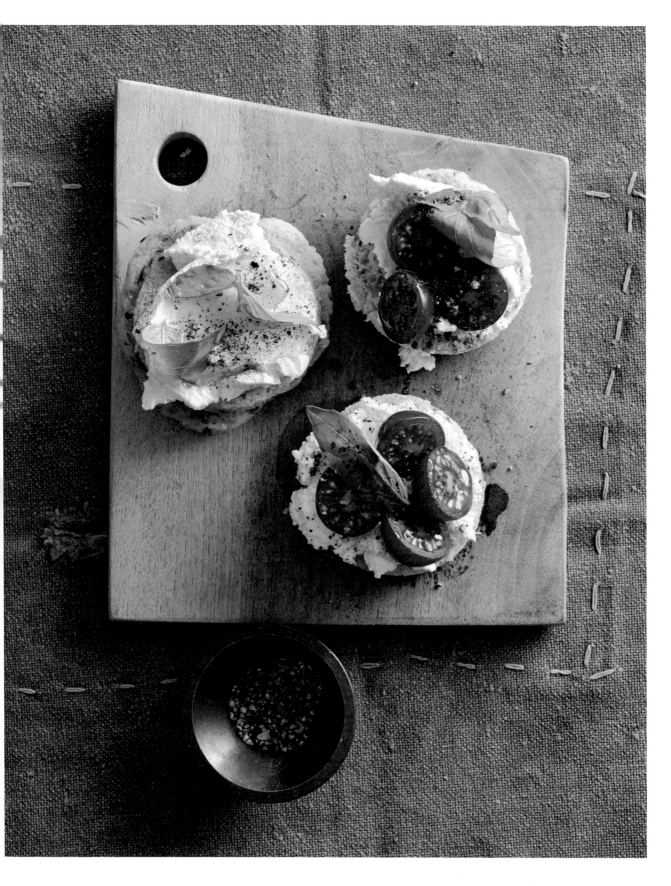

Quiche Lorraine

In this recipe, the pastry is the star of the dish – it crumbles and takes a savoury flavour from the Parmesan. Any extra can be cut into shapes and baked with the first baking of the quiche to make wonderful cheese biscuits. Vegetarians can make the pastry with butter and fill the quiche with the herb filling instead. Serve the quiche with the Green Salad on page 152.

Mix the pastry ingredients together by hand, crumbling the fat into the almonds, or use a food-processor. Once you have a smooth ball of pastry, flatten it a little to the size of your hand and wrap in clingfilm. Chill in the fridge for at least 30 minutes and up to a couple of days.

Preheat the oven to 200°C/fan 180°C/gas mark 6. Generously grease a 22cm (8½in) loose-bottomed tart tin.

Unwrap the pastry and roll out between two sheets of clingfilm to a thickness of 4mm (¼in). Lift into the tin and push the pastry gently into the grooves, neatening off the edges with a knife. Prick the bottom with a fork five times. Flatten any leftover pastry into biscuits about 5mm (¼in) thick and cook alongside the quiche for 10 minutes. Remove from the oven and set aside.

For the herb filling, whisk the herbs, cream and eggs together in a large bowl. Drop heaped teaspoons of the goat's cheese into the bowl and stir through.

For the bacon filling, gently sauté the onion and bacon in the fat for 8–10 minutes, or until the onion is translucent and the bacon is cooked through. Remove from the heat and set aside. Whisk the eggs and cream together in a large bowl. Stir in the cheese followed by the onion and bacon.

Pour the filling of your choice into the pastry case. Transfer carefully to a rack in the oven with a tray underneath. Bake for 20–25 minutes or until the crust is golden brown. Remove from the oven and set aside to cool for 15 minutes before removing from the tin and serving on a flat plate.

SERVES 8

For the pastry
45g (1¾oz) lard or butter, plus extra to grease
175g (6oz) ground almonds
1 tablespoon egg white (use the rest of the egg for the fillings)
25g (1oz) Parmesan, finely grated

For the herb filling
1 tablespoon thyme leaves, stalks discarded
3 tablespoons finely chopped chives
150ml (5fl oz) double cream
2 eggs and the remaining white and yolk
100g (3½oz) soft goat's cheese

For the bacon filling
1 small onion, finely chopped
10 rashers streaky smoked bacon, finely chopped
2 tablespoons extra virgin olive oil, lard or butter
2 eggs and the remaining white and yolk
150ml (5fl oz) double cream
75g (2¾oz) finely grated hard cheese (Cheddar, Comté, Parmesan, or a combination)

Per serving of herb quiche
2g carbs, 11.6g protein, 43g fat, 2.9g fibre, 362kcal

Per serving of bacon quiche
2.4g carbs, 11.3g protein, 43g fat, 2.9g fibre, 462kcal

Wraps

These versatile wraps are perfect for a quick bite or a packed lunch. They can also be used plain as chapati, as an alternative base to the pizza on page 82 or Flammekueche (page 76). The spices and herbs are optional flavourings, add or omit as you please.

Combine all the ingredients, except the fat, in a blender or use a whisk and bowl to make a smooth batter, adding your chosen flavouring (if using). Leave the batter to stand for 10 minutes. The batter can be made the day before and left in the fridge overnight. If it is very thick, dilute with a little more milk.

Warm the fat in a crepe pan or non-stick frying pan (about 22cm/8½in wide) over a medium-high heat and pour in 50ml (2fl oz) of the mixture. Tilt the pan or use a spatula to spread the batter out to form an even, round wrap. When golden brown on one side – usually after 3 minutes – flip the wrap over with a spatula and cook the other side until browned. Tip onto a plate and keep warm while you cook the remaining wraps. Usually after the first wrap I don't use any more fat, but add a little if they stick.

**MAKES APPROX.
6 X 15CM (6IN) WRAPS**

1 medium egg
40g (1½oz) buckwheat flour
30g (1oz) ground flaxseed
30g (1oz) ground almonds
270ml (9½fl oz) almond milk
¼ teaspoon salt
½ teaspoon cumin, pinch of chilli flakes, 1 teaspoon black onion seeds or a small handful of finely chopped coriander or parsley (optional)
1 teaspoon ghee, butter or extra virgin olive oil

Per wrap 6.5g carbs, 5.1g protein, 6.8g fat, 3g fibre, 113kcal

Fillings

TO FILL THE WRAP
Fill one edge of your wrap with a choice of filling ingredients and roll up. Cut in half at an angle and eat straight away. Alternatively, the wraps can be cooled and kept in the fridge, covered for a day or two. When cool, they can be filled and wrapped for a lunch on the go.
● Tahini Sauce, coriander and Italian Roasted Vegetables (page 144)
● Cream cheese and smoked salmon with either dill or parsley
● Mozzarella torn into pieces with roasted vegetables and basil leaves
● Hot fried eggs, crumbled feta, drizzle of extra virgin olive oil, coriander
● Torn cooked chicken, fresh tarragon, baby spinach, mayonnaise, lemon juice, freshly ground black pepper

TO MAKE THEM INTO FLATBREADS OR CHAPATI
Add chopped coriander and a few black onion or cumin seeds to the batter as you fry the wraps and top with a drizzle of extra virgin olive oil or ghee while still warm.

TO MAKE THEM INTO PIZZA
Top with 2 tablespoons Super Quick Tomato Sauce (page 90). Finish with torn mozzarella and basil leaves and bake for 5–7 minutes in a very hot oven.

Pizza

We all know that a good pizza is hard to beat. I have experimented with various alternative bases: cauliflower bases have an overpowering taste; cheese-only bases are just too fatty; and sweet potato bases are too high in carbs. So here we have it – ta-dah! Our perfect pizza base is made from the humble courgette and a handful of almonds. It is both crisp around the edges and supports the taste of the topping without overwhelming it – and the kids love it, too. I peel the courgette so that it doesn't have green flecks in the dough, but use the whole vegetable if you prefer.

Italy's "pizzaioli" (pizza-makers) are divided between those who prefer cow's milk mozzarella and those who would only dream of using buffalo milk mozzarella. The latter contains more water but, in my opinion, the taste is superior. If you choose to use cow's milk mozzarella, don't buy the one the manufacturers say is for making pizza – it is rubbery and flavourless. Just buy full-fat mozzarella. Whichever you opt for, tear the cheese into pieces and drain in a sieve while you make the bases.

Preheat the oven to 200°C/fan 180°C/gas mark 6. Line two baking trays with baking parchment and brush them with oil.

Put all the ingredients for the pizza base together in a bowl and mix with a large metal spoon. It will form a fairly thick dough.

Divide the dough into two and put a mound of the dough onto each lined tray. Press and shape each half with wet hands into a circle 1cm (½in) deep and 18–20cm (7–8in) in diameter. Bake for 10 minutes. Meanwhile, blend the ingredients for the tomato sauce together in a mixing bowl.

Remove the trays from the oven and slide the parchment onto the worktop. At this stage, the bases can also be cooled, wrapped tightly in clingfilm and kept in the fridge for 3 days or frozen for 3 months. Defrost before use. Put the oven trays back into the oven upside down to form a very hot, flat surface to cook the pizzas on. Increase the oven temperature as hot as it will go.

When you are ready to cook the pizzas, top each one with half the tomato sauce, leaving a finger-width border around the edge. Tear over the mozzarella and add the toppings you like. If you have a large cake slice, flat baking tray or flat wooden pizza peel, use this to move the pizzas onto the upturned trays.

Bake for 6–8 minutes until the mozzarella is bubbling and the crust becomes crisp and browned. Remove from the oven and serve with a drizzle of oil and the basil leaves.

MAKES 2 PIZZAS

For the base
extra virgin olive oil, to grease
25g (1oz) Parmesan
2 medium eggs
1 teaspoon salt
150g (5oz) ground almonds
1 medium courgette (approximately 175–220g/6–8oz), peeled and coarsely grated

For the tomato sauce
125g (4½oz) canned whole Italian plum tomatoes
1 teaspoon dried oregano
1 tablespoon extra virgin olive oil
¼ teaspoon salt
freshly ground black pepper

For the topping
75g (2¾oz) mozzarella, drained
A selection of the following
a handful of olives
8–10 slices of salami
8–10 slices of spicy chorizo
8 anchovies, drained from oil
thin strips of red pepper
2 spring onions, finely sliced
pinch of chilli flakes
extra virgin olive oil, to finish
a few basil leaves, to finish

Per serving with the tomato sauce and mozzarella but minus the further topping *9.8g carbs, 37g protein, 65g fat, 13g fibre, 647kcal*

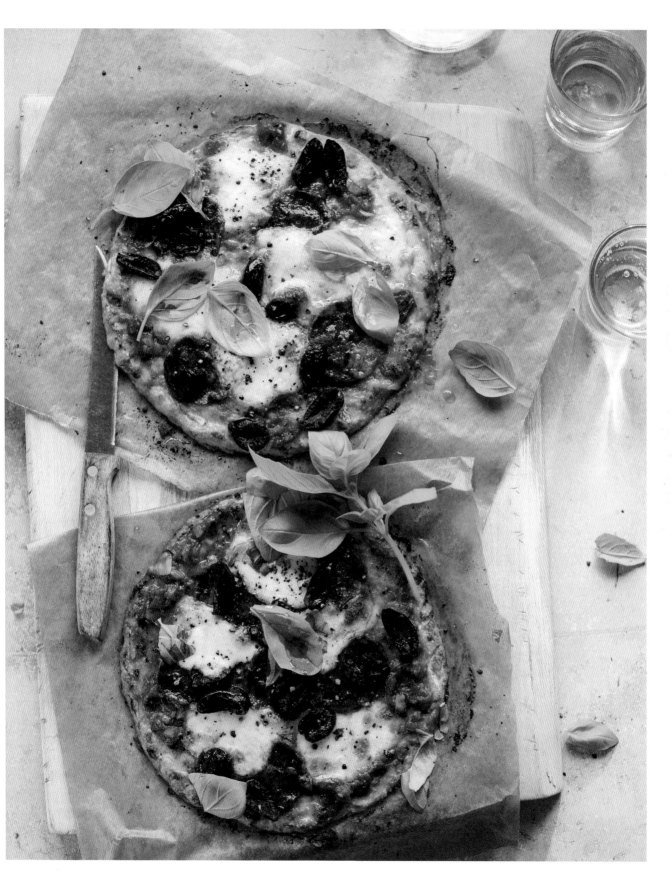

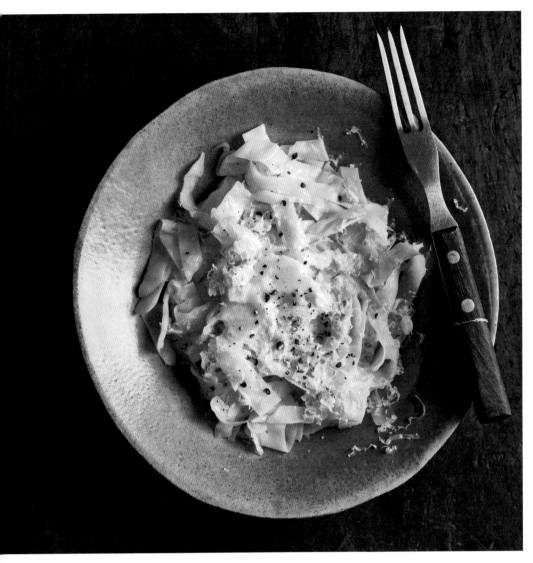

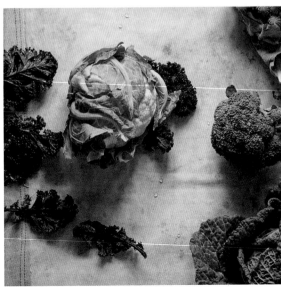

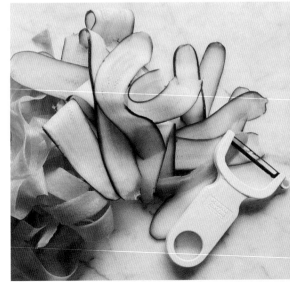

PASTA SAUCES *with everything but the pasta!*

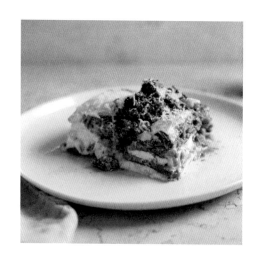

This chapter is devoted to alternatives to pasta to allow the enjoyment of all those wonderful pasta sauces we have cooked and served over the years, only this time without the carbs. In Giancarlo's case, since he is intolerant to gluten and carbs, his world of Italian food came crashing down and we had to think up other ways for him to eat the foods he loves. I remember giving him his first bowl of ragù on cabbage tagliatelle… I told him that it was a new type of pasta that was gluten-free – he loved it and has never looked back!

If you have type 2 diabetes or know that you are carb-intolerant, we recommend that you don't consume pasta. However, if you are in the medium to high end of the CarbScale, like Katie and personal trainer Natalia, the occasional bowl of pasta isn't going to hurt.

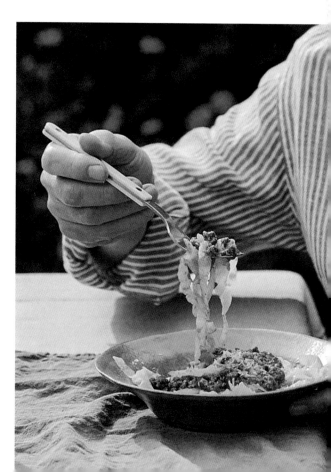

Asparagetti with Hot Smoked Salmon & Lemon Cream

Pale green ribbons of asparagus (we call them asparagetti) are the perfect, pretty partner for pink smoked salmon and a creamy white sauce.

Preheat the oven to 220°C/fan 200°C/gas mark 7.
Mix the asparagus ribbons with the oil, salmon and seasoning in an ovenproof serving dish and bake for 2–3 minutes until cooked through.

Meanwhile, warm the ingredients for the sauce in a large frying pan with a pinch of salt and pepper. As soon as the asparagetti is tender, splash over the sauce and serve straight away drizzled with a little extra oil.

SERVES 2

*200g (7oz) asparagus, shaved into
  ribbons (see below)
2 tablespoons extra virgin olive oil,
  plus extra to finish
200g (7oz) hot smoked salmon
  flakes or smoked salmon, roughly
  cut
salt and freshly ground black pepper*

For the sauce
*75ml (2½fl oz) double cream
2 tablespoons lemon juice*

Per serving *4.1g carbs, 29g protein,
41g fat, 1.7g fibre, 506kcal*

Roasted Root Ribbons

These colourful strands of root vegetables cook in just minutes in a hot oven and look stunning on a serving dish. Use a spiralizer with the thinnest slicer attachment, a sharp knife, potato peeler, mandolin or cheese slicer to create your ribbons; with a little practice you will find the best gadget to use. Try to serve a mixture of vegetables to vary the colour and flavour. These ribbons are robust enough for Beef Ragù (page 94) or are delicious served with roast meat, such as the Roast Pork Belly (page 114). To keep the carbs low, go for more celeriac and swede and less carrot and squash.

Preheat the oven to 200°C/fan 180°C/gas mark 4.

Toss the vegetable ribbons in a bowl with the oil and season. Add the thyme and lay on a baking tray in heaps and curls rather than flat so the heat can circulate easily.

Roast for 10–15 minutes until golden brown and tender. Remove the thyme sprigs and serve straight away.

SERVES 4

*400g (14oz) mixed vegetable ribbons
  cut from carrot, butternut squash,
  celeriac and swede
2 tablespoons extra virgin olive oil
few sprigs of thyme
salt and freshly ground black pepper*

Per serving *5.8g carbs,
0.9g protein, 6.6g fat, 3.1g fibre,
92kcal*

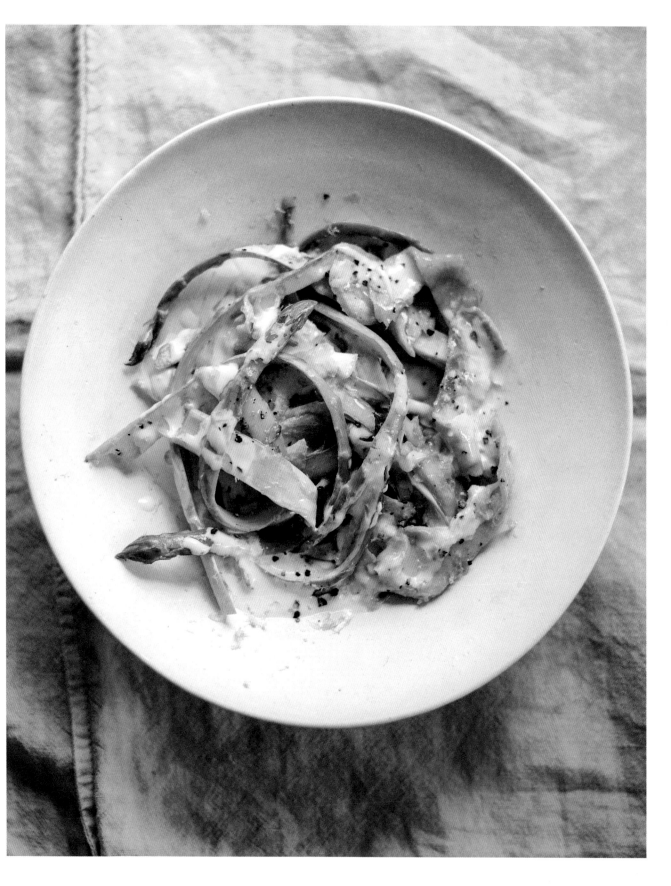

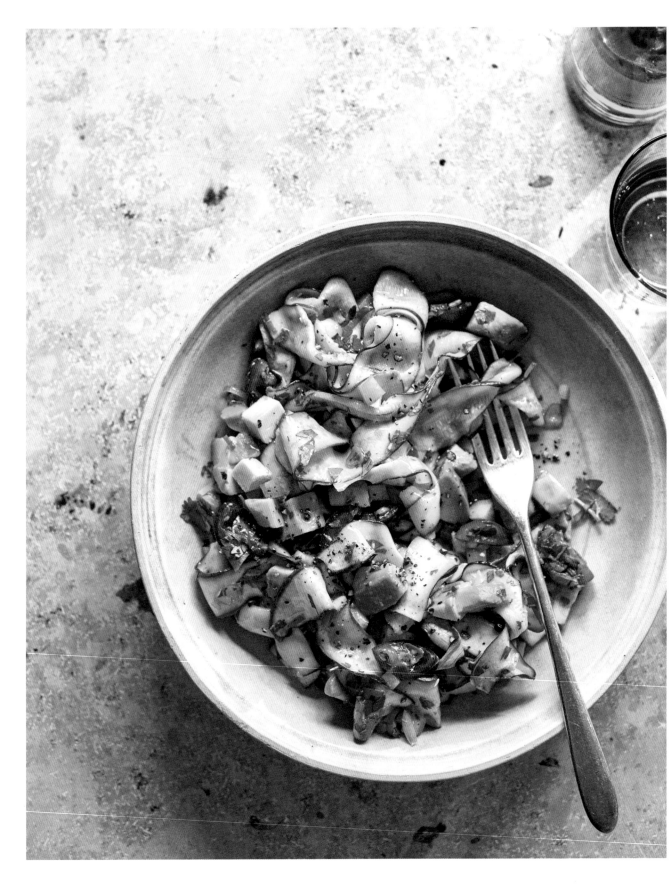

Courgette Ribbons with Avocado & Green Seasoning

This vegan dish is a rainbow in a bowl – we love its zing and freshness. Add tofu to bump up the protein or, if you eat meat and fish, try cooked chicken or fish.

Preheat the oven to 220°C/fan 200°C/gas mark 7. Line two baking trays with baking parchment.

Toss the ribbons in a bowl with the oil and season. Spread the ribbons out onto the baking trays in curls rather than flat so the heat can circulate easily. Bake for 2–3 minutes or until cooked through. Put into serving bowls and stir in the avocado, green seasoning, tomatoes and coriander.

SERVES 2

4 medium courgettes, made into ribbons (see page 86)
2 tablespoons extra virgin olive oil
1 large avocado, peeled, stoned and cubed
1 quantity Green Seasoning (page 138)
8 cherry tomatoes, quartered
a handful of coriander leaves
salt and freshly ground black pepper

Per serving *10g carbs, 8.6g protein, 37.5g fat, 10g fibre, 454kcal*

Cabbage Pappardelle

This is a really good alternative to ribbons of pasta such as pappardelle or tagliolini. White cabbage is firmer and will take a couple of minutes longer to cook to transform into soft, tender ribbons. It is perfect served with the Beef Ragù (page 94). Savoy cabbage is bright green and pretty when cooked and is excellent with pasta sauces.

Remove the hard core and outer raggedy leaves of the cabbage. Lay the cabbage flat side down and use a sharp knife to cut 1.5cm (⅝in) ribbons or very thin shreds.

Put the ribbons into a microwaveable bowl with the butter, a splash of water and some salt and pepper. Cover with clingfilm and microwave on full power for 5–7 minutes, stirring once halfway through.

Alternatively, put the cabbage ribbons into a medium saucepan with the butter, 100ml (3½fl oz) water and some salt and pepper, and cover with a lid. Cook over a medium heat for 8–10 minutes or until the ribbons are almost transparent and tender.

Drain before serving with the sauce of your choice.

SERVES 4

½ head of white or Savoy cabbage (approximately 500–700g/18oz– 1 lb 9oz)
10g (¼oz) salted butter
salt and freshly ground black pepper

Per serving *7.5g carbs, 1.8g protein, 2.2g fat, 4.5g fibre, 66kcal*

Super Quick Tomato Sauce

After years of not daring to alter Italian recipes from whichever mamma gave them to me, I have finally relented and made some changes to our tomato sauce recipe for when time is short. This sauce is very good if it is going to be cooked again, such as in the Aubergine Parmigiana (page 149) or Turkish Eggs (page 53).

Put all the ingredients together in a large frying pan and use a potato masher to break up the tomatoes. Bring the mixture to the boil, then reduce the heat so the sauce is bubbling rapidly. Cook for 10 minutes, stirring frequently, until the onion has softened and you are happy with the consistency. Leave the texture as it is or blend the sauce with a stick blender or in a food-processor.

For a **Classic Italian tomato sauce**, sauté the garlic and onions in the oil until soft, then add the tomatoes and cook for 40 minutes.

SERVES 6

5 tablespoons extra virgin olive oil
1 red onion, finely chopped
1 garlic clove, lightly crushed
  (optional)
2 x 400g (14oz) cans of Italian plum
  tomatoes
1 teaspoon salt
freshly ground black pepper

Per serving 7.1g carbs, 1.8g protein, 17g fat, 1.3g fibre, 196kcal

Roasted Vegetables with Tomato, Chilli & Cream Sauce

This is our new way to enjoy the spicy, creamy tomato sauce that we have been serving for 20 years in our restaurants. Instead of linguine we now love it on simple roasted vegetables.

Put the tomato sauce in a saucepan and add the chilli flakes and double cream. Heat gently until hot.

Serve the sauce poured over the roasted vegetables. Finish with some grated Parmesan, basil and a swirl of oil.

SERVES 2

1/3 quantity Super Quick Tomato
  Sauce or Classic Italian Tomato
  Sauce (see above)
good pinch of chilli flakes
2 tablespoons double cream
1 quantity Italian Roasted Vegetables
  (page 144)
25g (1oz) Parmesan, finely grated,
  to serve
a small handful of basil leaves,
  roughly torn
a swirl of extra virgin olive oil, to serve

Per serving 21g carbs,
7.8g protein, 47g fat, 9.3g fibre,
564kcal

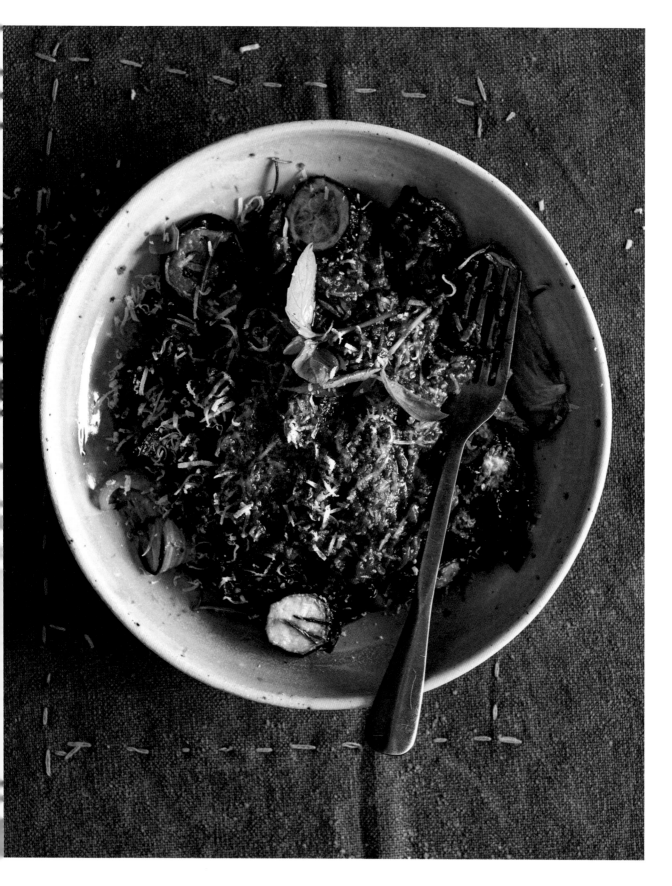

Cauliflower Pasta with Tahini Sauce & Hazelnuts

Small shapes of pasta, such as orrechiette (little ears), fusilli (spirals) or rigatoni (ridged tubes), are designed to trap the sauces served with them. However, if you are avoiding carbs, small florets of cooked cauliflower do the same job. We love this version with a Middle Eastern-inspired sauce using tahini. This vegan dish is filling and ticks all the boxes for a satisfying contrast of crunchy and soft textures in the same dish.

Preheat the oven to 220°C/fan 200°C/gas mark 7.

Put the nuts onto a baking tray and roast for 5–8 minutes or until lightly browned. Remove from the oven and lightly crush with a rolling pin or in a small food-processor. Keep them fairly chunky.

Put 3 tablespoons of the oil into a large frying pan over a medium heat. Add the spring onions, cauliflower and salt and pepper, and sauté with the lid on for 6–8 minutes, or until the cauliflower is just tender.

Remove the lid and allow any water to evaporate. Add the garlic and chilli and let them sizzle for a couple of minutes. Add the cumin and stir through.

Warm the milk and tahini together in a microwave or a small pan over a medium heat, whisking until smooth. Pour over the cauliflower in the pan and stir through.

Transfer to a warm serving dish or leave in the pan garnished with the nuts, a swirl of the remaining oil, the coriander and sesame seeds.

SERVES 2

50g (2oz) hazelnuts or walnuts
4 tablespoons extra virgin olive oil
3 spring onions or 1 shallot, finely chopped
250g (9oz) head of cauliflower, cut into bite-sized florets, with leaves, roughly chopped
1 garlic clove, finely chopped
1 small green chilli, finely sliced, or pinch of chilli flakes (according to taste)
1 teaspoon ground cumin
120ml (4fl oz) almond or cow's milk
3 tablespoons tahini
salt and freshly ground black pepper
a small handful of coriander leaves, to serve
1 teaspoon sesame seeds, to serve

Per serving *12g carbs, 14g protein, 59g fat, 7.7g fibre, 646kcal*

Ham Hock & Pea Risotto

Making a risotto from cauliflower rice is a great recipe for everyone; vegetarian or not, carb-intolerant or not. I have suggested adding a small amount of farro for texture – this is an ancient grain full of fibre and protein and low in gluten. It is higher in carbs than cauliflower, but it's good for the very active among us. Use lower-carb quinoa or omit it completely, depending on where you are on the CarbScale. By cooking and then cooling the farro, you are increasing the resistant starch, and therefore reducing the absorbed carbohydrate.

Start by cooking the farro, spelt or quinoa (if using) following the instructions on the packet. Once cooked through, drain and tip into a bowl (add a splash of oil if it looks sticky) and leave to cool.

Heat the oil and half the butter in a large, heavy-based frying pan over a medium heat. Sauté the bacon (if using), leek, celery, garlic, rosemary and thyme for 5–7 minutes or until the leek is soft.

Increase the heat to medium, add the cauliflower rice to the pan and fry, stirring constantly with a wooden spoon, for a few minutes. Add the ham hock and farro, spelt or quinoa (if using) to the pan and stir through, then pour in the wine. Bring to the boil and cook for 4 minutes before adding the stock, a little at a time, to create the loose consistency of a risotto. The amount of stock will differ if you have used farro, spelt or quinoa. Cook for a further 5–7 minutes or until the cauliflower is tender.

Steam the peas for 2 minutes and add to the pan with the remaining butter, the cream and Parmesan. Stir through. Season to taste. Spoon the risotto into warmed bowls and serve scattered with parsley.

SERVES 6

50g (2oz) farro, spelt or quinoa (optional)
3 tablespoons extra virgin olive oil
50g (2oz) salted butter
100g (3½oz) ham hock or 4 rashers, streaky smoked bacon, finely sliced
1 leek or white onion, finely chopped
1 celery stick, finely chopped
1 fat garlic clove, lightly crushed
1 sprig of rosemary
3 sprigs of thyme
1 small head (approximately 600g/1lb 5oz) of cauliflower and leaves, riced (see page 166)
100ml (3½fl oz) white wine
300ml (10fl oz) vegetable stock, Chicken Stock (page 203) or hot water
50g (2oz) sugar snap peas, finely sliced, or frozen peas
75ml (2½fl oz) double cream or crème fraîche
75g (2¾oz) Parmesan, finely grated
a small handful of parsley, roughly chopped
salt and freshly ground black pepper

Per serving with farro 15g carbs, 13g protein, 25g fat, 3.3g fibre, 347kcal
Per serving without farro 9.6g carbs, 12g protein, 25g fat, 2.8g fibre, 319kcal

Variation

MUSHROOM & PEA RISOTTO
Omit the bacon for a vegetarian option. Sauté 500g (18oz) sliced portobello or chestnut mushrooms in a separate pan with 4 tablespoons of extra virgin olive oil and salt and pepper. Fry for 10–15 minutes until the mushrooms are lightly browned. Add to the pan with the leek and celery when they are soft. Continue as above.

Beef Ragù

This is a rich and utterly delicious beef ragù – there is always some in our fridge. It is a sauce I have been making for the last 20 years since I married into an Italian family. The only difference is that instead of having it with pasta, we now eat it with Cabbage Pappardelle (page 89), Italian Roasted Vegetables (page 144), eggs cooked in the heat of the ragù or in the Tuscan Lasagne on page 100. Do try and find coarsely minced meat that has around 15 per cent fat in it; the fat will add flavour and prevent the ragù from becoming dry. The vegetables can be cut into tiny pieces in a food-processor, but be careful that you don't end up with a purée.

Heat the oil in a large saucepan and fry the garlic, carrot, celery, onion and bay leaves for about 15 minutes, or until softened.

Meanwhile, put the tomatoes into a bowl and break them up a little with your hands or with scissors. Rinse out the empty cans with a splash of water and add this to the bowl.

Add the minced meat to the pan and fry until browned, breaking it up with a wooden spoon. Any water in the mince should come out at this point, so only add the red wine when you see the minced meat starting to look dry. Let it reduce for 5 minutes.

Add the tomatoes, bring the ragù to the boil, then immediately reduce the heat to a gentle simmer. Leave for at least 2 hours, adding a little more water if the ragù starts to look dry (though this shouldn't be necessary if it is only just simmering).

Remove the bay leaves and serve straight away, or leave to cool and store in a covered container in the fridge for up to a week, or freeze for up to 3 months.

**SERVES 8/
MAKES 1.2KG (2LB 12OZ)**

80ml (3fl oz) extra virgin olive oil
2 garlic cloves, lightly crushed
1 medium carrot, very finely chopped
2 large celery sticks, very finely chopped
1 red onion, very finely chopped
2 bay leaves
2 × 400g (14oz) cans of Italian plum tomatoes
850g–1kg (1lb 14oz–2¼lb) minced beef, veal or pork, or a mixture
200ml (7fl oz) red wine

Per serving 6.4g carbs, 29g protein, 13g fat, 1.5g fibre, 272kcal

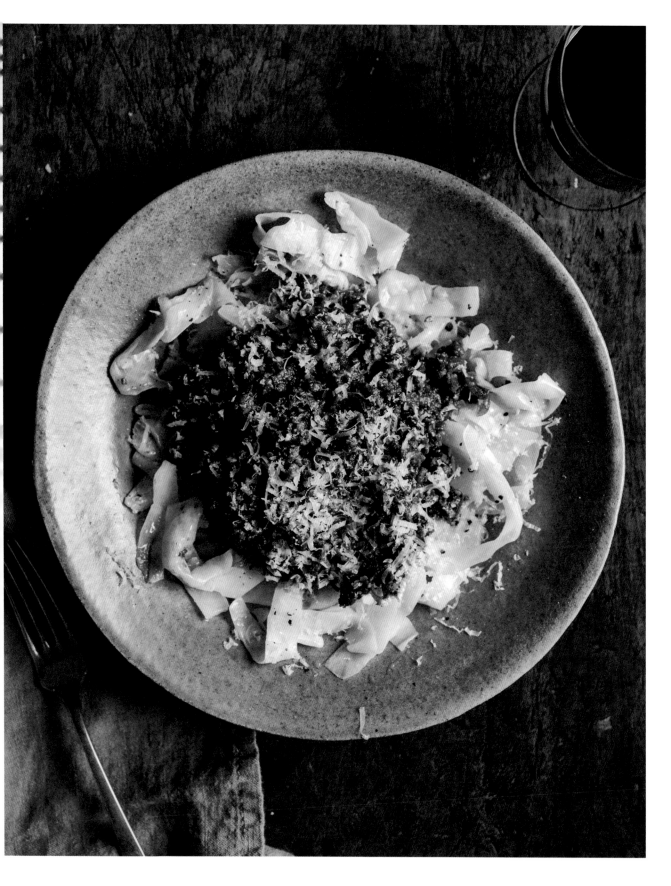

Mushroom "Pasta" Rotolo

We are very proud of this alternative to pasta created with mushrooms and egg, but the real genius is the psyllium husk powder – a natural binder that allows vegetables and egg to become a pasta-like sheet strong enough to use for lasagne, cannelloni or even cut into tagliatelle.

Preheat the oven to 220°C/fan 200°C/gas mark 7. Line a baking tray with baking parchment and brush with a little oil. Set aside.

To make the mushroom pasta, sauté the mushrooms in the oil with a pinch of salt and a good twist of black pepper over a high heat until the water has evaporated and they have begun to sizzle and stick. Stir frequently with a wooden spoon. Remove from the heat and leave to cool for a few minutes.

Once cooled, blitz in a food-processor to form a paste and then add the eggs, milk and psyllium husk powder. Blitz again until very smooth and no visible pieces of mushroom remain.

Spread the mushroom mixture onto the lined tray. Put another piece of oiled baking parchment over the top and carefully press it out to form a thin rectangle measuring roughly 27 x 34cm (10¾ x 13¼in) and about 5mm (¼in) thick. Remove the top piece of parchment. Tidy it up as necessary and even it out with a flat-ended tool, such as a fish slice or dough scraper.

Bake for 8–10 minutes or until it is firm to the touch and set through. Remove from the oven and leave to cool on the tray.

To make the filling, toss the vegetables in the oil with the thyme, season with salt and pepper, and roast on a baking tray for 20–25 minutes or until tender and lightly browned. Remove from the oven and set aside to cool for 15 minutes.

Spread half of the tomato sauce onto the mushroom pasta, leaving a border of 1cm (½in) around the edge. Scatter over the hard cheese, the roasted vegetables and most of the basil leaves, leaving a handful for the end. Using two dessertspoons drop heaped dollops of mascarpone over the surface until it is used up.

Roll up the rotolo on the paper from the long edge to form a long Swiss roll. Use the paper to pull the roll towards you. Spread half of the remaining tomato sauce on a lasagne dish long enough to hold the rotolo. Using your hands, carefully transfer the rotolo to sit on top of the tomato sauce. Top with the remaining tomato sauce.

Bake for 20 minutes. Remove from the oven and leave to rest for 10 minutes, before serving scattered with the remaining basil leaves.

MAKES 1 SHEET (enough for 1 rotolo)/SERVES 4

3 tablespoons extra virgin olive oil, plus extra to grease
250g (9oz) mushrooms, brushed clean and roughly sliced
2 eggs
2 tablespoons almond or cow's milk
1 heaped teaspoon psyllium husk powder
salt and freshly ground black pepper

For the filling
1 red pepper, diced into 2cm (¾in) cubes
1 medium courgette, diced into 2cm (¾in) cubes
2 tablespoons extra virgin olive oil
few sprigs of thyme or ½ teaspoon dried oregano
1 quantity Super Quick Tomato Sauce (page 90)
100g (3½oz) smoked hard cheese or Cheddar, coarsely grated
a large handful of basil leaves
150g (5oz) mascarpone

Per serving *14g carbs, 18g protein, 66g fat, 7.7g fibre, 741kcal*

Spinach "Pasta"

We usually use bags of frozen spinach for this. They are sold in 900g–1kg (2–2¼lb) bags and, to give you a guide, 900g (2lb) of frozen spinach becomes 300g (10½oz) once it is defrosted and squeezed well. Don't buy chopped spinach if you have the choice as it is harder to squeeze.

These sheets are ideal to use as an alternative to the mushroom pasta in our Mushroom "Pasta" Rotolo (see opposite) or cut them into rectangles and use for the Tuscan Lasagne (page 100). The mushroom and spinach "pasta" sheets can be rolled around oiled baking parchment and covered with clingfilm and either kept refrigerated for up to 3 days or frozen for 3 months.

Preheat the oven to 220°C/fan 200°C/gas mark 7. Line two baking trays with baking parchment and grease with the olive oil.

Blitz the ingredients together in a food-processor to form a paste. Spread the mixture evenly onto the lined trays. Put another piece of oiled baking parchment over the top of each and carefully press out to form two thin rectangles measuring roughly 27 × 34cm (10¾ × 13¼in) and about 5mm (¼in) thick. Remove the top sheet of paper. Tidy up as necessary and even out with a flat-ended tool, such as a fish slice or dough scraper.

Bake for 8–10 minutes or until firm to the touch and set through. Remove from the oven and leave to cool on the tray.

MAKES 10–12 LASAGNE SHEETS
cut into rectangles measuring approx. 9 × 13cm (3½ × 5in)
SERVES 6

extra virgin olive oil, for greasing
370–400g (13–14oz) defrosted spinach, squeezed from a 900g (2lb) bag of frozen spinach
½ teaspoon salt
4 eggs
8 tablespoons almond or cow's milk
1 heaped tablespoon psyllium husk powder

Per serving *0g carbs, 7.2g protein, 4.2g fat, 4.5g fibre, 77kcal*

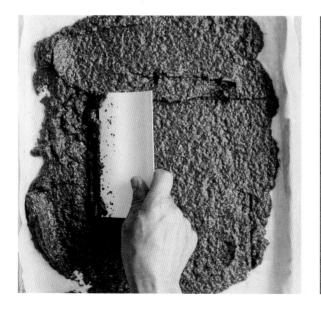

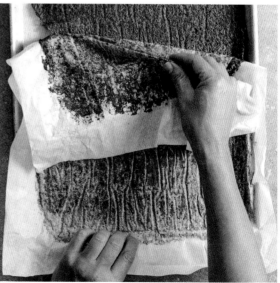

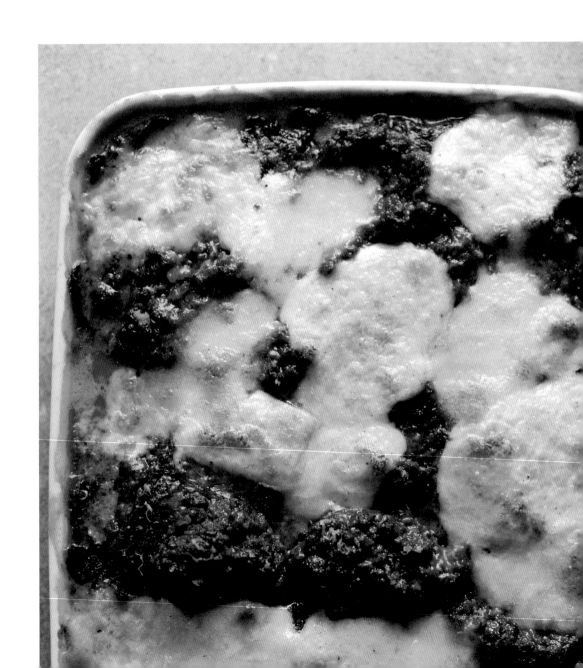

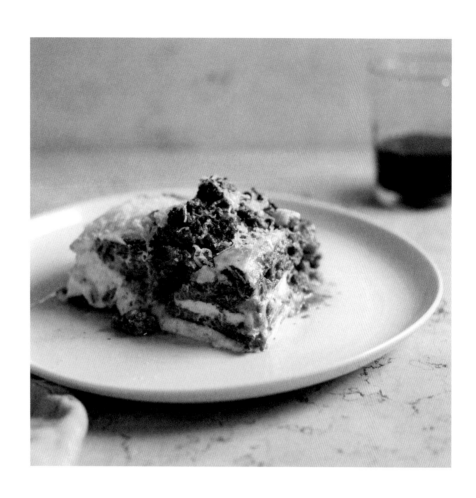

Tuscan Lasagne

This is Giancarlo's mother's recipe. I am not quite sure what she would make of our spinach pasta, but I know her son loves it and it doesn't raise his blood sugar levels! It has become the new lasagne in the house and is loved by all. The kids barely noticed that the pasta vanished – it tastes and looks just as gorgeous as their grandmother's.

Preheat the oven to 200°C/fan 180°C/gas mark 6.

To make the béchamel, mix 3 tablespoons of the milk with the cornflour in a small bowl. Pour into a saucepan with the remaining sauce ingredients and put over a medium heat. Whisk to combine and remove from the heat once it has thickened and is bubbling. Season to taste.

Using a dessertspoon, drop spoonfuls of a quarter of the béchamel and ragù on the base of a lasagne dish measuring approximately 22 × 26cm (8½ × 10½in). Don't mix them together. Now scatter over a quarter of the Parmesan and mozzarella.

Cut the spinach pasta into shapes to fit your dish. It could be in one single sheet, rectangles or other shapes, but try not to have too much overlapping. Lay a third of the pasta over the béchamel and ragù.

Follow this sequence until you have three layers of pasta and four layers of béchamel, ragù and cheese.

Bake for 30 minutes. Let the lasagne sit and settle for at least 15 minutes before enjoying.

SERVES 6

1 quantity Béchamel (page 139)
700g (1lb 9oz) Beef Ragù (page 94)
50g (2oz) Parmesan, finely grated
125g (4½oz) mozzarella, roughly torn
1 quantity Spinach "Pasta" (page 96)

For the béchamel
(Makes approx. 650g/1lb 7oz)
550ml (19fl oz) almond or cow's milk
4 tablespoons cornflour
4 tablespoons double cream
50g (2oz) butter
½ teaspoon salt
¼ teaspoon freshly grated nutmeg
1 bay leaf

Per serving *3g carbs, 25g protein, 16g fat, 5.1g fibre, 270kcal*

Mushroom Lasagne

Follow the instructions for the Tuscan Lasagne (opposite), but replace the ragù with the mushroom mixture below.

Preheat the oven to 240°C/fan 220°C/gas mark 9 or as hot as your oven will go.

Toss the mushrooms in a large bowl with the remaining ingredients and a good twist of pepper. Put them onto two baking trays spread out into single layers so the heat can get to all of them. Roast for 15–20 minutes, or until lightly browned. Remove from the oven and leave to cool to room temperature before using for the lasagne (see opposite).

SERVES 6

1kg (2¼lb) chestnut mushrooms, brushed clean and finely sliced
5 tablespoons extra virgin olive oil
1 onion, finely chopped
2 garlic cloves, lightly crushed
2 sprigs of thyme
1 sprig of rosemary
½ teaspoon salt
freshly ground black pepper

For whole recipe 42g carbs, 27g protein, 65g fat, 10g fibre, 837kcal
Per serving 21g carbs, 20g protein, 39g fat, 6.6g fibre, 515kcal

Variation

ROASTED VEGETABLE LASAGNE
Follow the instructions for the Tuscan Lasagne, but replace the ragù with the Roasted Vegetables on page 144 and mixed with either of the tomato sauces on page 90.

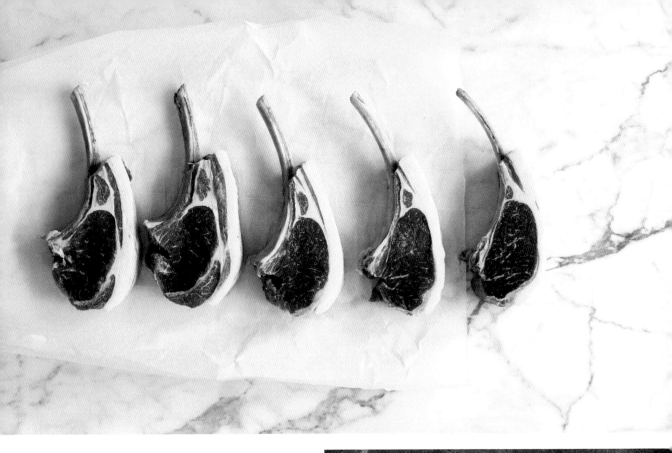

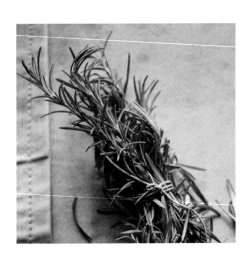

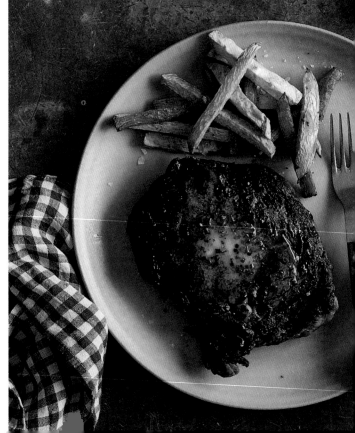

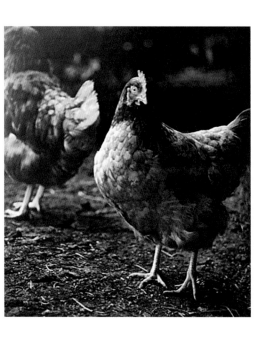

MEAT *and* POULTRY

Meat, glorious meat! Despite my former life as a vegetarian I now have to admit my huge pleasure in being carnivorous. I lost my vegetarianism on an Italian train as I was seduced by a panino stuffed full of layers of fatty, salty, pink Parma ham. I have never looked back, but I do try to feed our family a varied diet of good-quality meat, fish and plenty of vegetarian food as well.

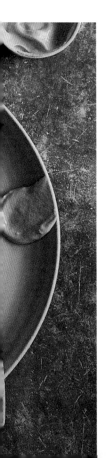

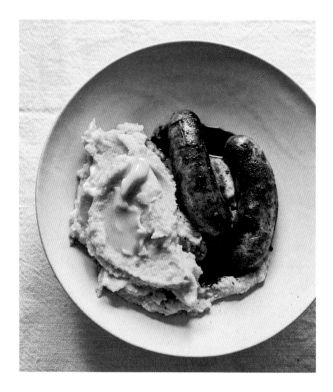

Lamb & Halloumi Kebabs

This is the ultimate fast food as the kebabs take just 3 minutes to cook on each side. The lemony marinade introduced to us by our friends Sandie and Peter Draper stops the meat from drying out. These can be done under a hot grill if you don't have glowing coals outside. Serve the kebabs with lettuce wraps and a bowl of the Lemon Yogurt Sauce.

To make the marinade, put all the ingredients into a small food-processor with a good few twists of pepper and blend until emulsified. Alternatively, you can chop the dry ingredients together finely by hand and mix with the oil.

Pour a third of the marinade into a shallow dish with the lamb, peppers, mushrooms and onion, and toss to combine. Cover and leave to infuse for at least 30 minutes and up to a day in the fridge. Put the remaining marinade into a jug and refrigerate.

To make the lemon yogurt sauce, mix the ingredients together in a bowl and season to taste. This will keep in the fridge, covered, for up to 3 days.

When you are ready to cook the kebabs, preheat the grill to high and heat a rack ready for the kebabs. Thread the lamb, peppers, mushrooms, onion and halloumi alternately onto metal kebab skewers. Discard any leftover marinade in the dish.

Lay the skewers onto a hot grill rack (if this is in an oven, put an oven tray underneath to catch the juices) and cook close to the heat source for 3–4 minutes before turning and cooking again for 3 minutes, or until the cheese is browned and the meat is just cooked. These are also delicious barbecued.

Put the lettuce leaves and the bowl of lemon yogurt sauce on a large serving dish. Add the hot skewers dressed with a little of the remaining marinade and sprinkled with parsley. Serve the remaining marinade in a jug.

SERVES 8

For the marinade
150ml (5fl oz) extra virgin olive oil
4 garlic cloves, peeled
½–1 medium hot red chilli (according to taste)
1 x 20cm (8in) sprig of rosemary
½ teaspoon chilli flakes
6 sprigs of thyme (leaves picked)
2 bay leaves
finely grated zest and juice of 1 lemon
1 teaspoon salt
freshly ground black pepper

For the kebabs
600g (1lb 5oz) lean lamb (leg meat is good), diced into 3cm (1¼in) cubes
2 red peppers, cut into 3cm (1¼in) squares
250g (9oz) small chestnut mushrooms, brushed clean
1 red onion, cut into quarters and layers separated
2 x 250g (9oz) halloumi, cut into bite-sized cubes
3 baby gem lettuces, leaves separated, to serve
1 quantity Lemon Yogurt Sauce (see below), to serve
a small handful of parsley, leaves coarsely chopped and stems finely chopped, to serve

For the lemon yogurt sauce
8 tablespoons Greek yogurt
8 tablespoons mayonnaise
finely grated zest of 1 lemon
salt and freshly ground black pepper

Per serving 8g carbs, 33g protein, 65g fat, 2.1g fibre, 755kcal

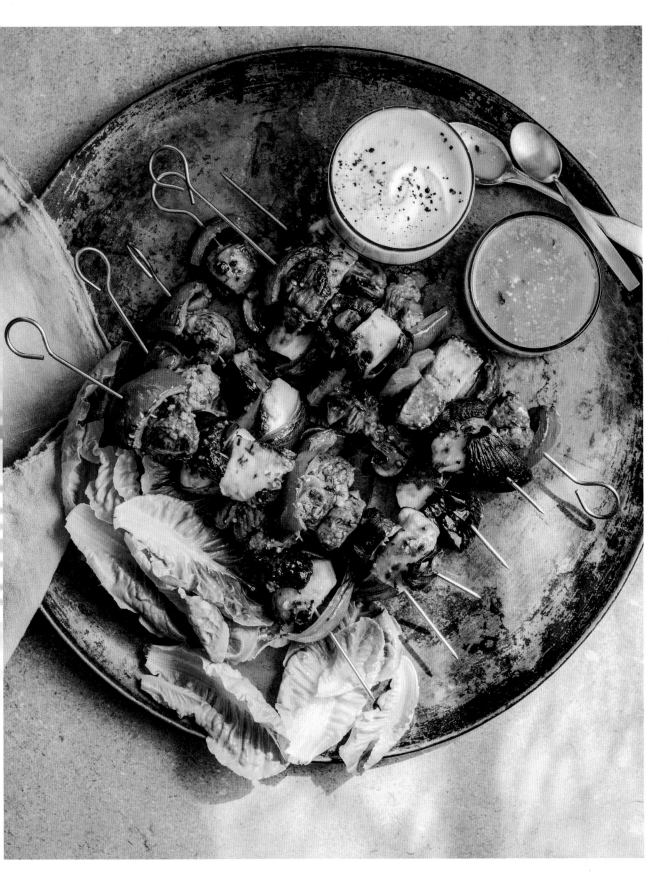

Aubergine "Little Shoes"

This has all the traditional flavours of Greek moussaka without the frying and faff of making the layers. Halved and roasted aubergines are used to hold the spicy lamb and cheese topping, called "little shoes". To make the filling into an Italian lamb ragù rather than Greek moussaka, leave out the cinnamon and oregano.

Preheat the oven to 220°C/fan 200°C/gas mark 7.

Make diagonal shallow cuts in the surface of each aubergine half and lay them onto a baking tray. Brush with half the oil and season with salt and pepper. Bake for 35– 40 minutes, or until the flesh is cooked through and lightly browned.

Meanwhile, heat the remaining oil in a pan and soften the onion and garlic over a medium heat for 7–10 minutes. Add the minced lamb and break it up with a wooden spoon as it browns. Add the cinnamon and oregano.

When the lamb has browned all over and most of the water from the meat has evaporated, pour in the wine. Reduce for 5 minutes before adding the tomatoes. Add 100ml (3½fl oz) water to the can, swirl it round and add this, too. Continue to cook over a low heat for 1 hour, stirring frequently. Taste and add more seasoning if necessary.

When the aubergines are soft, remove them from the oven and push the centres down with a metal spoon to create cavities to stuff with the lamb.

Reduce the oven temperature to 200°C/fan 180°C/gas mark 6. Spoon off any excess oil from the lamb. Fill the aubergine "shoes" with the lamb mixture, dividing it equally between them.

Mix together the ingredients for the topping so that it is well blended. Season with salt and pepper and pour it on top of the aubergines. Bake for 20–25 minutes or until the cheese topping is golden brown. Serve.

SERVES 6

For the lamb filling
4 aubergines, halved lengthways
7 tablespoons extra virgin olive oil
1 medium onion, finely chopped
3 garlic cloves, lightly crushed
500g (18oz) minced lamb
1 teaspoon ground cinnamon
1 teaspoon dried oregano
125ml (4fl oz) red wine
1 x 400g (14oz) can of plum
  tomatoes
salt and freshly ground black pepper

For the topping
50g (2oz) Parmesan, finely grated
2 large eggs
175ml (6fl oz) full-fat Greek yogurt
¼ teaspoon ground nutmeg

Per serving 9.3g carbs, 25g protein, 34g fat, 4.6g fibre, 468kcal

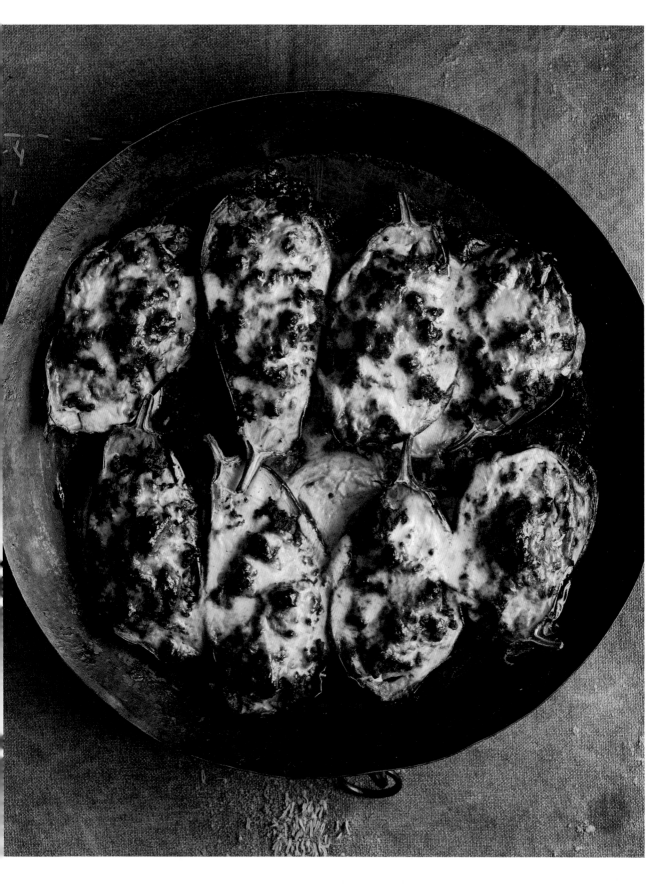

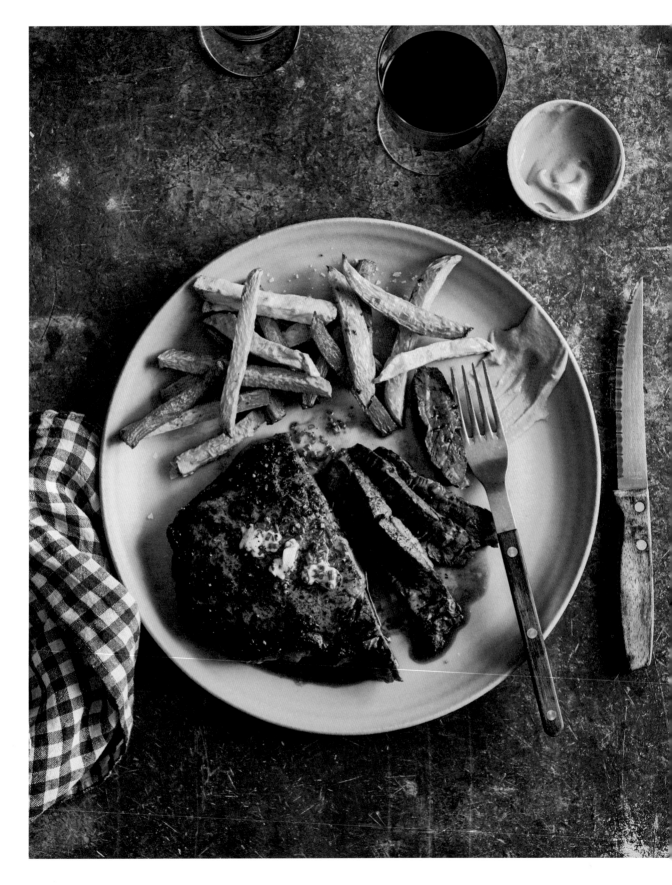

Steak with Herb & Garlic Butter

On our cooking courses, many people ask why their steak doesn't taste like those cooked in a restaurant. Apart from the quality of the meat and hanging time, it is the fact that the hand of a chef will be more generous with the salt than that of a home cook. It's as simple as that!

   This steak is delicious served with shards of herb and garlic butter and, instead of potatoes, have our Chips (page 171), Roasted Root Ribbons (page 86) or Celeriac Dauphinoise (page 171) alongside it. Now butter is back on our menu, we love to mix it with flavourings and watch shards of it melt onto hot steak or fish, spread it onto warm low-carb bread (page 69), or stir it into mash or mushrooms. Basil is my favourite flavour, while Giancarlo loves garlic, rosemary and black pepper. Chives, parsley, fresh oregano or tarragon are gorgeous, too.

To make the herb butter, mix the ingredients together in a bowl, adding plenty of black pepper, and use a spatula to shape the butter into a shallow rectangle about 1cm (½in) deep on a piece of baking parchment. Cover with more parchment and put in the fridge (or the freezer if you are in a hurry) to firm up before using.

Bring the steaks to room temperature. Massage a generous pinch of salt and some pepper into each steak just before cooking.

Heat the fat to very hot in a frying pan, then add the seasoned steaks and cook until the steaks are done to your liking (see box below).

Ideally, cooked meat should be rested for the same amount of time as it takes to cook. This is because when meat is cooked the juices move to the inside of the meat, causing the outside to be dry. Allowing meat to rest means the juices are evenly distributed again.

We like to serve steak "tagliata", which means cutting the steak into finger-width strips, topped with the herb butter.

SERVES 4

4 sirloin or ribeye steaks
   (approximately 200–250g/
   7–9oz each)
2 tablespoons beef dripping, goose fat
   or chicken fat
salt and freshly ground black pepper

For the Herb & Garlic Butter

60g (2¼oz) salted butter, at room
   temperature
6g (¼oz) finely chopped herbs
1 small garlic clove, grated (optional)
freshly ground black pepper

Per steak 0g carbs, 64g protein,
37g fat, 0g fibre, 587kcal

As a guide, a sirloin steak 2cm (¾in) thick will take 1½ minutes per side for rare; 2 minutes per side for medium-rare; and 3 minutes per side for medium. To tell when a steak is ready, press the top of it while it is still in the pan or under the grill. The resistance to your touch will demonstrate how it is cooked. You can compare the feeling to various parts of your hand, using this simple guide:

● Press your thumb and index finger together and prod the soft fleshy area at the base of your thumb with the index finger of your other hand. It will be soft to the touch like a "rare" steak feels.
● Move your middle finger to touch your thumb and feel the point again – it will feel like a "medium-rare" steak.
● The third finger will make it feel like "medium".
● The little finger will make it feel like "well done".

Meat Patties with Tomato Chilli Jam

In our quest to find different versions of this recipe we have made kofte in Kuwait; reindeer and moose burgers in Lapland; meatballs in tomato sauce in Italy and Greece; and spicy reshmi in India. It seems most cultures have worked out that patties made from minced meat taste pretty darn good.

We have used spinach instead of breadcrumbs to give the patties colour, texture and moisture, but you can omit the spinach, if you like – the result will be a slightly firmer patty. It's best to use 10 per cent fat minced meat, rather than the lean version, to add juiciness and flavour.

These patties are great to make in batches. They will keep in the fridge, covered, for up to 4 days, or can be frozen, so are good for quick meals.

Sakis Kalliontzis from Cooking Workshop Consulting – a cookery school in Thessaloniki – introduced me to this chilli jam recipe. It is an excellent substitute for sugary chilli jam or tomato ketchup and it's even popular with my teenagers, so it has to be good! It is great to make when you have a lot of very ripe, squishy tomatoes. Use one variety or blend a few together.

To make the tomato chilli jam, put all the ingredients into a large frying pan and bring to the boil. Reduce the heat to medium and continue to cook for 20 minutes, stirring frequently.

Remove from the heat and leave to cool a little. Tip into a bowl or a liquidizer (reserve the pan) and blend until smooth.

Pour back into the pan and reduce to a thick ketchup consistency. This will take 10–15 minutes. Taste and adjust the seasoning as necessary. Serve warm or leave to cool and store in a sealed jar in the fridge for up to 5 days.

To make the patties, combine all the ingredients for the patties in a bowl, cover with clingfilm and, as my Greek cookery teacher Sakis said, "Leave it to have a siesta in the fridge for 30 minutes!" for the flavours to combine.

Preheat the oven to 220°C/fan 200°C/gas mark 7. Grease a baking tray.

To check for seasoning, take a walnut-sized amount of the mixture, flatten it to a patty and dry-fry it in a small, non-stick pan until browned and cooked through. Taste and adjust the seasoning or spices as you like.

Make up the remaining patties (making eight in total) and lay onto the prepared tray. Bake on a rack over a baking tray for 15 minutes or until cooked through. They can also be fried in lard, chicken fat, ghee or extra virgin olive oil for 6–8 minutes, turning them once during that time. Serve hot with the tomato chilli jam, Greek yogurt and salad.

SERVES 4/MAKES 8 PATTIES
approx. 50g (2oz) each
or 4 patties approx.160g
(5¾oz) each

*100g (3½oz) defrosted and
    squeezed dry spinach, finely
    chopped (from 300g (10½oz)
    frozen spinach)
500g (18oz) minced lamb, venison,
    beef or pork, or a mixture
1 small onion, finely chopped or
    coarsely grated
2 garlic cloves, finely grated
1½ teaspoons salt
freshly ground black pepper*

**For the Tomato Chilli Jam (Makes
approx. 270g/9¾oz)/SERVES 10**
*400g (14oz) tomatoes (cherry, round,
    plum), tough green cores removed,
    roughly chopped
1 x 400g (14oz) can of plum
    tomatoes or passata
1 teaspoon salt
few sprigs of thyme
½ teaspoon ground cinnamon
¼–½ teaspoon chilli flakes, added
    according to taste
½ teaspoon dried oregano
freshly ground black pepper*

Per serving of patties *2.3g carbs,
25g protein, 14g fat, 235kcal*
Per serving of tomato chilli jam
*2.7g carbs, 0.6g protein, 0g fat,
0.7g fibre, 19kcal*

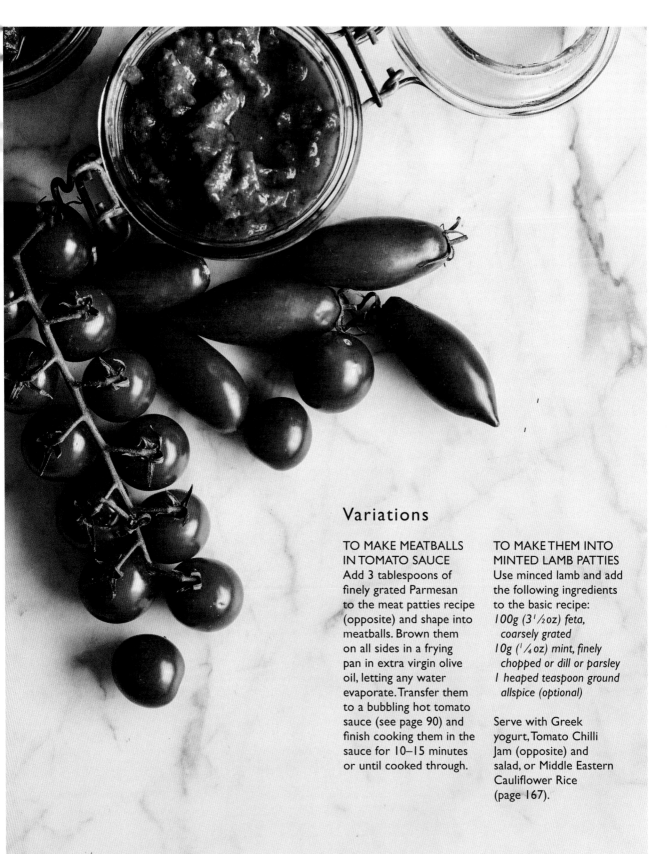

Variations

TO MAKE MEATBALLS IN TOMATO SAUCE

Add 3 tablespoons of finely grated Parmesan to the meat patties recipe (opposite) and shape into meatballs. Brown them on all sides in a frying pan in extra virgin olive oil, letting any water evaporate. Transfer them to a bubbling hot tomato sauce (see page 90) and finish cooking them in the sauce for 10–15 minutes or until cooked through.

TO MAKE THEM INTO MINTED LAMB PATTIES

Use minced lamb and add the following ingredients to the basic recipe:

100g (3 1/2 oz) feta, coarsely grated
10g (1/4 oz) mint, finely chopped or dill or parsley
1 heaped teaspoon ground allspice (optional)

Serve with Greek yogurt, Tomato Chilli Jam (opposite) and salad, or Middle Eastern Cauliflower Rice (page 167).

Indian Beef Patties

This is based on our friend Nina Powar's recipe for reshmi. These are delicious served with Indian Cauliflower Pilao (page 166) or Mango & Avocado Salad (page 119). If you aren't keen on coriander, substitute it for dill, parsley or mint. This is a real cheat's dip and is perfect with any of the curries in the book (see pages 117 and 163). Decorate with a little mint or black onion seeds if you have them.

Preheat the oven to 220°C/fan 200°C/gas mark 7. Soak 12 wooden skewers in cold water for 30 minutes.

Blend all the paste ingredients together in a small food-processor or finely chop by hand to form a coarse paste. Put into a bowl with the meat patties mixture, mix together with your hands, cover with clingfilm and leave to marinate for 30 minutes in the fridge.

To make the dip, combine the ingredients together in a bowl and set aside until ready to serve.

Once chilled, press about 60g (2¼oz) of the mixture firmly onto each of the soaked wooden skewers. Cook on a grill rack above a tray in the oven for 13–15 minutes or until cooked through. They are also delicious barbecued. Serve the patties with the dip.

SERVES 6/MAKES approx. 12 skewers

1 quantity Meat patties mixture (page 110)

For the paste
30g (1oz) fresh ginger, peeled
2 garlic cloves, peeled
20g (¾oz) coriander leaves
2 small green chillies
2 teaspoons ground cumin
1 tablespoon garam masala, or meat masala powder
1 teaspoon hot paprika, unsmoked, or chilli powder
1 teaspoon ground turmeric

For the Yogurt & Lime Pickle Dip
250g (9oz) Greek yogurt
2 tablespoons lime pickle from a jar, finely chopped

Per serving of yogurt dip
2.4g carbs, 2.5g protein, 5.2g fat, 0g fibre, 67kcal

Beef Bone Broth

Good stock or "bone broth", has been the remedy for ill health for centuries as the collagen in the stock helps to soothe the stomach as well as the soul. Broth is good to drink while fasting as it fills you up until the next meal. Jenny's tip is to freeze the broth in a silicone muffin moulds then gather them together in a bag and just take one out as needed. Defrost one in a mug, heat and add hot water to the top with fresh ginger and coriander.

Preheat the oven to 220°C/fan 200°C/gas mark 7. Put the bones, carrots, onion and celery into a roasting tin and roast for 1 hour. Halfway through, toss everything together. Remove from the oven and use tongs to transfer the bones and vegetables into your largest pot. Reserve the fat for future use.

Add the remaining ingredients and top up with cold water to cover the bones. Bring to the boil, then reduce the heat to a very gentle simmer. Cook for around 12 hours. Allow to cool before straining and storing.

MAKES 1–2 LITRES (1¾–3½ PINTS)

2.5kg (5½lb) beef bones
4–5 litres water
2 carrots, roughly chopped
1 large white onion, cut into quarters (don't bother to peel it)
2 celery sticks, roughly chopped
a few celery leaves
a few parsley stalks
1 bay leaf
150ml (5fl oz) red wine

Per 100ml serving *carbs, 3.7g protein, 4.6g fat, 0g fibre, 61kcal*

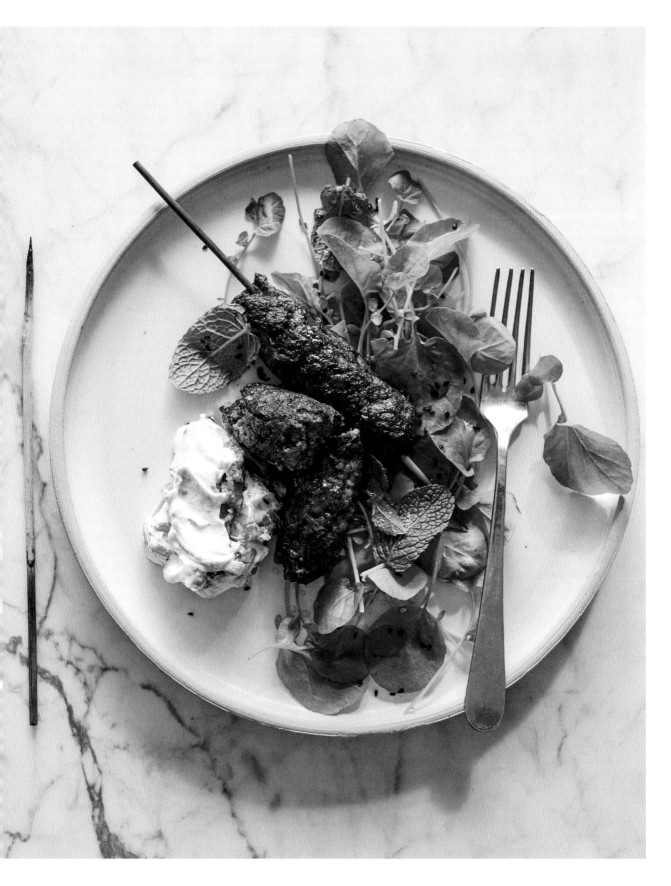

Roast Pork Belly & Stuffed Onions

This roast pork has a crisp, crunchy crackling that looks fabulous and works each time thanks to our chef friend Laurence Keogh and our local butcher Devin from Savannah. The trick is to open the pores of the skin to let the salt in, which draws out the water making excellent crackling. Ask your butcher to score the skin in diagonal lines a finger width apart or do it yourself with a Stanley knife. Any colour of onion works but they should be short and fat so that they can sit upright to hold the filling. Serve the pork with Roasted Root Ribbons (page 86).

Preheat the oven to 260°C/fan 240°C/gas mark 9. Lay the pork belly, skin-side up, in a roasting tin. Pour over a kettleful of boiling water. The skin will whiten and swell. Then carefully pour the water away. Repeat once more. Pat the belly dry thoroughly with kitchen paper and rub the salt into the skin. Leave to rest for 10 minutes before drying again.

Blend the stuffing ingredients together in a food-processor to form a paste. Spread this evenly onto the inside of the pork belly. Roll the belly up and tie with butcher's string to keep it in a roll. Put it onto a rack over a roasting tin.

To make the stuffed onions, pour the salt into a large baking dish and stand the unpeeled onions on the salt, tops pointing up. Wrap the dish tightly in foil.

Place the pork in the centre of the oven and roast for 40–50 minutes, or until the skin is blistered all over, then remove from the oven. At the same time, bake the onions for 40 minutes. Reduce the temperature to 170°C/fan 150°C/gas mark 3. Tip away the fat in the roasting tin or save for roasting vegetables.

Return the pork to the oven on a clean tray and cook for 1½–2 hours until tender inside. Test by pushing a sharp knife into the flesh on one end. If there is a lot of resistance, leave it a little longer. Remove the foil from the onions and bake for a further 30 minutes. Remove from the oven and leave to cool.

Once cool, cut off the top third of each onion and discard the tops. Scoop out the centre with a spoon, leaving two layers of flesh and the base intact. If you spot a hole in the bottom of any, cover it with a small piece of the scooped-out onion. Purée the scooped-out onion with the cheese and oil in a food-processor or chop finely by hand. Season to taste. Fill each onion shell with purée and put back on top of the salt. Scatter with a little more cheese and bake for 15–20 minutes until browned and bubbling.

To make the jus, put all the ingredients into a saucepan and bring to the boil. Reduce the heat to medium and let the sauce reduce by half. Season to taste. Pass the sauce through a fine sieve into a gravy boat and keep warm. When the pork is cooked, remove from the oven and allow to rest for 20 minutes. Remove the string and serve with the onions and jus.

SERVES 10

1 boneless pork belly (approx. 2½–3kg/5½–6½lb 8oz–6lb 8oz)
3 teaspoons fine salt

For the stuffing
50g (2oz) pine nuts
25g (1oz) sage leaves
2 fat garlic cloves, peeled
50ml (2fl oz) extra virgin olive oil
1 heaped teaspoon salt
freshly ground black pepper

For the stuffed onions
300g (10½oz) coarse salt
6 small–medium brown or red onions (they should all be the same size)
75g (2¾oz) Parmesan or Pecorino, finely grated, plus extra to serve
3 tablespoons extra virgin olive oil
salt and freshly ground black pepper

For the jus
500ml (18fl oz) Chicken Stock (page 115)
500ml (18fl oz) Beef Bone Broth, (page 112) or beef stock
50ml (2fl oz) tomato juice or passata
2 shallots, finely chopped
200ml (7fl oz) red wine
sprig of fresh thyme
1 bay leaf
1 garlic clove, lightly crushed

Per serving of pork belly
0.6g carbs, 64g protein, 51g fat, 0g fibre, 716kcal
Per serving of stuffed onions
0g carbs, 4.4g protein, 10g fat, 0g fibre, 109kcal
Per serving of jus 0.7g carbs, 3.1g protein, 2.7g fat, 0g fibre, 55kcal

Chicken & Something Soup

I loved my mother's chicken soup; she learned to be frugal during the war and always added the cooked chicken picked from the carcass. She collected the fat from roasting and used it for cooking. I have carried on both traditions. Instead of thickening soup with potato, we use Brussels sprouts (the "something"), which give the soup body. Fresh or leftovers can be used, and if you have any sprout haters, just don't tell them what's in the soup – it is puréed so no one will know!

Sauté the onions or leeks, celery, herbs and seasoning in the fat over a medium heat for 7–10 minutes, or until softened.

Add the sprouts and stir through. Sauté for a further 5 minutes before adding the stock. Bring to the boil, reduce the heat and simmer for 15 minutes.

Once the vegetables are cooked, purée the soup with a stick blender or liquidizer to a smooth consistency, taking care the hot soup doesn't splash you.

Heat the soup in the pan and add the cooked chicken. Warm to bubbling, then serve in bowls with the parsley, some black pepper and a swirl of oil.

SERVES 6–8

3 tablespoons chicken fat, extra virgin olive oil, ghee or butter
2 onions or 2 leeks, finely chopped
2 large celery sticks, finely chopped
2 sprigs of thyme
1 sprig of rosemary
300g (10½oz) Brussels sprouts, trimmed and roughly chopped
2 litres (3½ pints) warm Chicken Stock (page 203)
200g (7oz) cooked chicken, torn into bite-sized pieces
a handful of parsley, finely chopped
extra virgin olive oil
salt and freshly ground black pepper

Per serving 4.8g carbs, 15g protein, 7.8g fat, 2g fibre, 154kcal

Chicken Stock

Making chicken stock reminds me of my childhood as my mother would always make it on a Monday after we had a roast chicken. She would pick the meat from the carcass keeping it to add to other meals. Do hunt down chicken sold with giblets if you can; it makes all the difference. If you are using cooked carcasses and bones, skip the roasting stage.

Preheat the oven to 220°C/fan 200°C/gas mark 7. Put the carcasses into a roasting tin with the vegetables and roast for 1 hour.

Remove from the oven and use tongs to transfer the bones and vegetables to a stock pot with the giblets (if using). Pour any remaining fat into a bowl for use another time.

Deglaze the tin with the white wine and tip this into the pot. Pour over 5 litres (8¾ pints) of cold water and bring to the boil. Add the bay leaf and Parmesan rind (if using). Reduce the heat to a very gentle simmer and cook for at least 3 hours and up to 6 hours.

MAKES 3–4 LITRES
(5¼–7 PINTS)

2–3 raw chicken carcasses
1 white onion, cut into eighths
2 large celery sticks plus any leaves, roughly chopped
1 carrot, halved
200ml (7fl oz) white wine
1 bay leaf
1 Parmesan rind (optional)

Per 100ml (3½fl oz) serving
1.1g carbs, 3.7g protein, 4.6g fat, 0g fibre, 61kcal

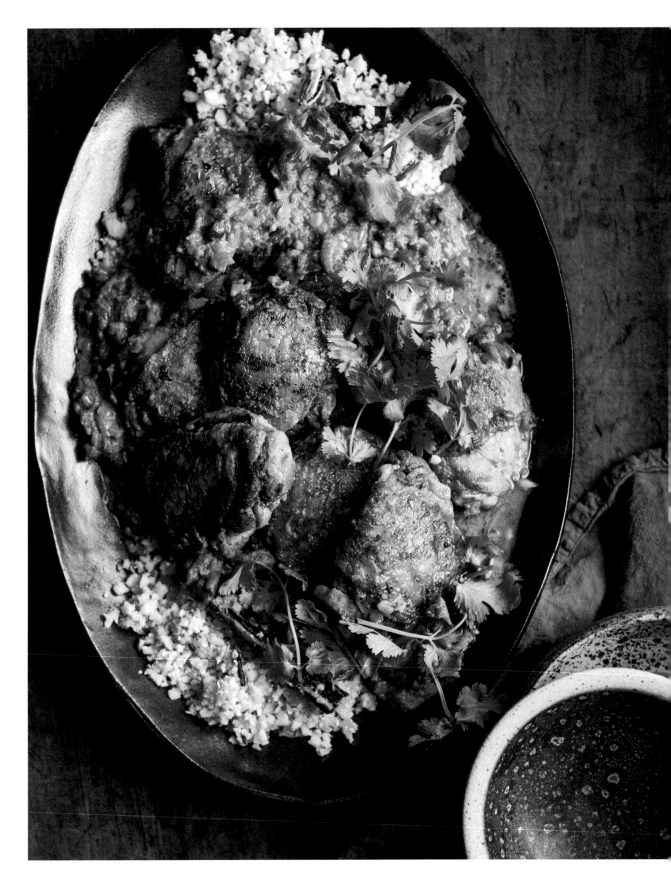

Butter Chicken

We love this creamy, golden curry that delivers a spicy punch in a velvet glove. It is easy to make and doesn't have the sugar or commercial oil that a takeaway contains. It can be made in advance and kept in the fridge or freezer. Use breast meat if you prefer it to thighs and cut the cooking time down accordingly. The sauce can be left as it is or blended. Serve with the Indian Cauliflower Pilao on page 166 or the Lentil-less Dal on page 164, yogurt and lemon wedges.

Put the chicken thighs into a bowl and scatter over 1 flat teaspoon of salt, the chilli powder, lemon juice and half the garlic and ginger. Mix thoroughly and set aside to infuse for 15 minutes.

Put the chicken thighs skin-side down into a large frying pan over a medium heat. When golden brown turn to the other side and repeat – it will take aabout 20 minutes to do this. Remove the chicken from the pan and set aside while you make the sauce.

Add the ghee to the pan (unless there is enough remaining chicken fat) and fry the onion with a little salt until softened – this will take about 10 minutes.

Add the remaining garlic, ginger and chilli and fry for a couple of minutes. Stir in the spices and cook for another couple of minutes.

Add the butter and tomatoes and fill the can halfway with water and swirl it around, add this to the pan and cook for 15 minutes, or until the tomatoes are soft, stirring frequently. Add the thighs to the pan and continue to cook, covered with a lid, for 45 minutes or until they are cooked through and the meat falls easily from the bones. Season to taste. Add the coriander and serve straight away.

SERVES 4

8 chicken thighs, skin on and bone in
salt
2 teaspoons chilli powder
2 tablespoons lemon juice
4 fat garlic cloves, grated
1 tablespoon fresh ginger, peeled and grated
2 tablespoons ghee, butter or coconut oil (optional)
2 onions, finely chopped
1–2 small green or red chillies, split in half, added according to taste
2 teaspoons ground cumin
1 teaspoon ground turmeric
1 teaspoon ground coriander
50g (2oz) butter
1 x 400g (14oz) can of plum tomatoes, chopped
a few coriander leaves

Per serving 10g carbs, 67g protein, 60g fat, 2.5g fibre, 857kcal

Kuwaiti Spiced Lamb Shoulder with Yogurt & Mint Sauce

This is based on a recipe shown to us by our Kuwaiti friend Amal Al Alquatani. It is very easy to put the dish together and the lamb becomes meltingly soft and tender. This is perfect served with Yogurt & Mint Sauce (see below) and Middle Eastern Cauliflower Rice (page 167).

Preheat the oven to 240°C/fan 220°C/gas mark 7. Allow the lamb to come to room temperature to ensure it cooks evenly.

Prepare the stuffing by blending all the ingredients together using a small food-processor or chop by hand.

Make five deep cuts in the lamb on the top and bottom and push a little of the stuffing inside each one. Smear the rest of the stuffing all over the lamb and lay it into a roasting tin. Pour 150ml (5fl oz) cold water around the lamb and then cover the whole tray with two sheets of foil, wrapping it underneath the tin to ensure the steam will stay inside.

Roast for 20 minutes. Reduce the oven temperature to 180°C/fan 160°C/gas mark 4 and roast for a futher 2¾ hours.

To make the sauce, mix the ingredients together in a bowl. Season to taste. Finish with a swirl of oil and some black pepper. Transfer to the fridge to chill before serving.

Remove the lamb from the oven and carefully remove the foil, being careful of the steam. To test if the meat is done, pull the shoulder bone away slightly. The meat around it should give easily. If it is not done to your liking, replace the foil and return the lamb to the oven (this can happen if the shoulder is very large).

Once cooked, remove the lamb from the tin and transfer to a warmed serving dish. Cover with foil and a couple of cloths to keep it warm and allow to rest for 20 minutes before serving. Carve, and serve with the sauce.

SERVES 8

2kg (4½lb) lamb shoulder

For the stuffing
6 garlic cloves, grated
40g (1½oz) fresh ginger, peeled and grated
75g (2¾oz) butter
1 tablespoon thyme leaves
1 teaspoon ground turmeric
2 teaspoons ground cinnamon
2 teaspoons ground cumin
2 teaspoons salt
freshly ground black pepper

For the yogurt & mint sauce
300ml (10fl oz) Greek yogurt
a large handful of mint, leaves picked and finely chopped
1 garlic clove, finely grated
2 tablespoons extra virgin olive oil, plus extra to finish

Per serving 2.7g carbs, 38g protein, 44g fat, 0g fibre, 559kcal

Very Simple Chicken Tikka with Mango & Avocado Salad

Garam masala and masala powders are spice blends that save time. However, the taste does differ between brands – my reliable favourite is Everest, available online or at Asian shops. Some masala powders contain salt so do taste it first. The recipe works wonderfully with salmon, too and is delicious with Yogurt & Lime Pickle Dip (page 112). This tropical salad was shown to me by our personal trainer Natalia Giers, and is good with curries, chicken or grilled fish.

For the paste, blend the ginger, garlic, chilli, spices and salt together in a small food-processor to form a paste and then stir in the yogurt. If you don't have a small food-processor, grate the ginger and garlic and finely chop the chilli instead.

Pour the paste over the chicken in a container and stir through to coat it. Leave to marinate, covered, for at least 30 minutes or overnight in the fridge.

To make the salad, put the avocado, mango, chilli and leaves in a serving bowl.

To make the salad dressing, mix the oil, lime juice, black onion seeds and seasoning together in a small bowl and pour over the salad just before serving. Use tongs to gently combine the fruit, leaves and dressing.

Preheat the grill to high.

Thread the pieces of chicken onto metal skewers leaving a little gap between each one. Lay the skewers onto a grill rack over a baking tray. Grill near to the source of heat as they look and taste better when lightly browned. Turn once during the cooking time and check they are cooked through – this will take 8–10 minutes. If you have a meat thermometer, check that the chicken is 80°C (176°F) inside, or cut into the deepest part with a sharp knife to check that the juices run clear and are not pink. Don't overcook the chicken as it will dry out. The skewers are also delicious barbecued. Serve the skewers with the salad.

SERVES 6

1kg (2¼lb) boneless, skinless chicken breast, cut into 5cm (2in) cubes

For the paste

15g (½oz) fresh ginger, peeled
5 garlic cloves, peeled
1 small hot green or red chilli or ½ teaspoon chilli flakes (added according to taste)
¼ teaspoon unsmoked paprika
1 tablespoon masala powder
½ teaspoon salt
150g (5oz) Greek yogurt

For the Mango & Avocado Salad

1 large ripe avocado, peeled, stoned and diced into 2cm (¾in) cubes
1 slightly unripe mango, peeled, stoned and diced into 2cm (¾in) cubes or sliced
1 big green mild chilli or green pepper, finely sliced
200g (7oz) rocket, baby spinach or watercress, roughly torn
4 tablespoons extra virgin olive oil
juice of 2 limes
1 teaspoon black onion seeds
salt and freshly ground black pepper

Per serving 5.9g carbs, 3.5g protein, 16g fat, 2.8g fibre, 185kcal

Thai Green Curry

This spicy, creamy curry will fill you up without piling on the pounds if you don't have it with rice. Either eat it as a soup from a bowl or enjoy it with Southeast Asian Cauliflower Rice (page 167). You can substitute the chicken for pork, beef, salmon or prawns. Traditionally, coriander root is used, but since this can be hard to source we use the stems instead. Since the paste keeps well when frozen, we normally make twice the amount and freeze half for another day.

Use a food-processor to blitz the paste ingredients to a smooth consistency. Use straight away, store in a sealed container in the fridge for up to 3 days, or freeze in bags for up to 3 months.

To make the curry, heat the fat in a wok or large frying pan and fry the paste until it releases its fragrance – about 2 minutes. Add the coconut milk, the stock or water (if cooking thighs) and the chicken and bring to the boil. Reduce the heat and simmer for up to 45 minutes or until the chicken is cooked through (breast meat will take 15–20 minutes). Season to taste.

Stir in the spinach leaves and then serve in warm bowls scattered with basil.

SERVES 6/MAKES 400g (14oz) curry paste

For the Thai Green Curry Paste
1 teaspoon Thai shrimp paste or fish sauce (optional)
4–5 green Bird's Eye chillies, roughly chopped (according to taste)
4 dried Kaffir lime leaves or 1 fresh Kaffir lime leaf, roughly chopped
1 finger galangal or fresh ginger, peeled and roughly chopped (approx. 40g/1½oz)
2 lemon grass stalks, chopped
3 garlic cloves
½ teaspoon salt
50g (2oz) fresh coriander (roots if you have them, stems and leaves), roughly chopped
1 white onion, chopped
1 teaspoon ground coriander
1 teaspoon ground cumin
½ teaspoon white pepper (or black if you don't have white)

For the curry
1 tablespoon coconut oil, chicken fat or extra virgin olive oil
1 quantity Thai Green Curry Paste (see above)
1 x 400g (14oz) can of coconut milk
150ml (5fl oz) hot Chicken Stock (page 115) or water (if you are cooking thighs)
700g (1lb 9oz) bone-in chicken thighs, skinned, or breast meat, roughly chopped
500g (18oz) baby spinach leaves, washed
a handful of Thai sweet basil or Italian basil, shredded

Per serving 6.3g carbs, 34g protein, 25g fat, 2.3g fibre, 392kcal

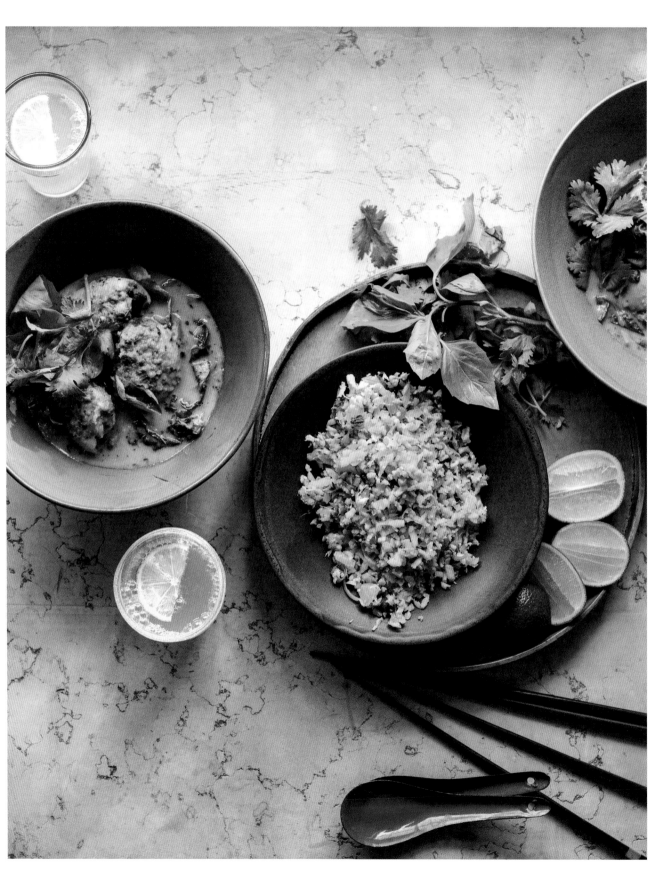

Flavio's Warm Chicken & Pesto Salad with Crackling

Our son Flavio loves to cook. This is his way of serving hot, juicy chicken, crispy skin and freshly-made pesto. Try to find chicken thighs without the bones but with the skin on. Alternatively, leave the bones in and cook for about 15 minutes longer to ensure the chicken is cooked through.
The pesto will make more than you need for this recipe, but you can keep it in the fridge for up to 5 days and use it on the Courgette Ribbons (page 89), on salmon, or swirled into any of the mash recipes (pages 170).

Preheat the oven to to 220°C/fan 200°C/gas mark 7. Put the pine nuts on a baking tray and roast for a few minutes until golden brown. Remove from the oven and tip onto a plate to cool.

Peel the skin from the chicken thighs and set aside. Season the thighs lightly with salt and pepper and stretch each one out onto a baking tray.

Now stretch out the pieces of skin onto an oven rack, scatter with a little salt and cook just above the chicken thighs in the oven for about 25 minutes, the fat from the skin will drip onto the thigh meat below. The skin will shrink and become golden and crispy and the chicken thighs should be cooked through in about the same time, but do remove one or the other if one is ready before.

Meanwhile, to make the pesto, whizz all the ingredients together in a small food-processor or use a pestle and mortar. Season to taste and set aside.

When the chicken is cooked, remove the rack with the skin and set aside. Remove the tray with the chicken thighs and spoon over the pesto, using about 1 tablespoon per thigh. Tear the mozzarella into thumb-sized pieces and lay on top of the pesto. Scatter the tomato halves around the chicken and bake for a further 5 minutes or until the cheese begins to brown.

To make the salad, toss the spinach with the oil and a pinch of salt and pepper, and divide between four bowls or plates. Lay the chicken onto the spinach with the tomatoes, crumble the chicken crackling over the top and serve.

SERVES 4

8 boneless chicken thighs, skin on
125g (4¼oz) mozzarella
16 cherry tomatoes, halved
salt and freshly ground black pepper

To make the pesto (serves 8)
125g (4½oz) pine nuts
50g (2oz) basil leaves and stalks
25g (1oz) Parmesan, finely grated
1 small garlic clove, peeled
125ml (4fl oz) extra virgin olive oil

For the salad
200g (7oz) spinach leaves
1 tablespoon extra virgin olive oil

Per serving of chicken salad
3g carbs, 34g protein, 25g fat,
2.7g fibre, 385kcal
Per serving of pesto 1g carbs,
3.9g protein, 26g fat, 0.6g fibre,
257kcal

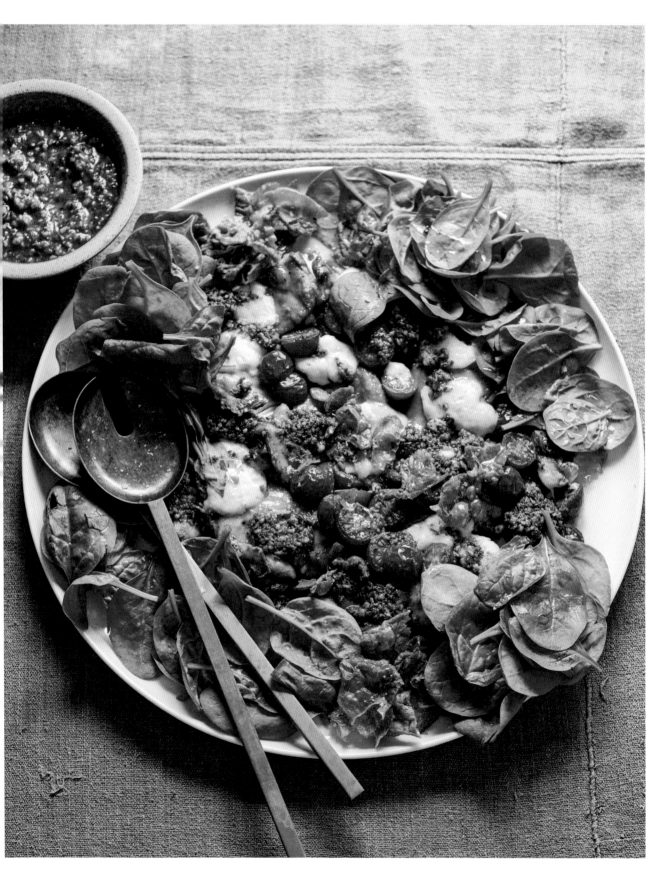

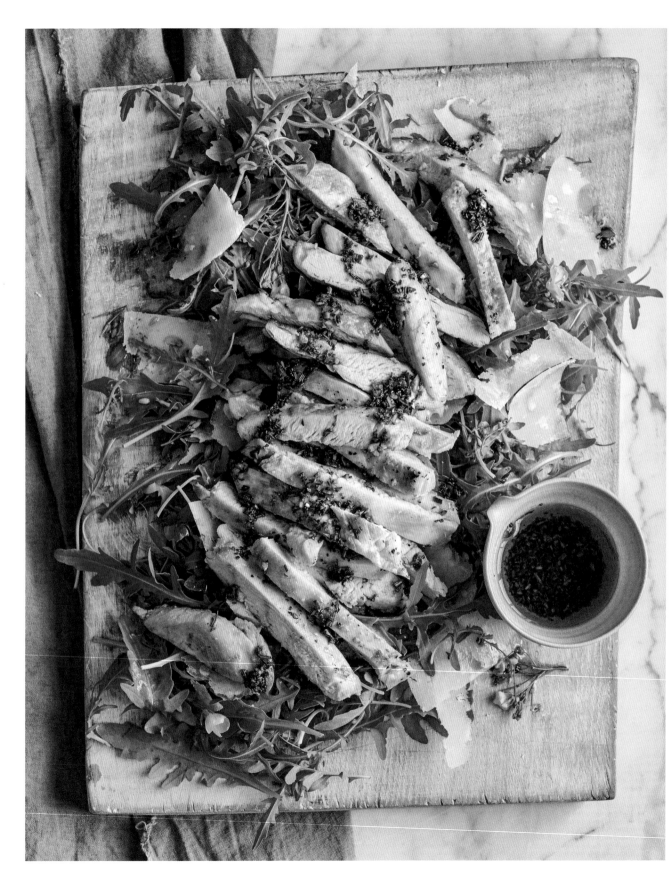

Chicken Tagliata

Tagliata means "cut" in Italian and refers to the fact that the chicken is cut into strips while hot to allow the unctuous spicy dressing to soak in. This recipe comes from Gino Borella who was Head Chef of San Lorenzo in Knightsbridge for 30 years. He cooked thousands of dishes for so many famous people over the years, including Princess Diana, and this was one of her favourites. The dressing keeps for up to a week in the fridge. If you have chicken skin, cook it as per the recipe on page 122 and crumble it over the top.

Preheat the grill to high.

Prepare the dressing by finely chopping the rosemary, chilli and garlic together on a board with some salt and a good twist of pepper. Mix in a small bowl with the oil and vinegar. Set aside.

Open out the chicken breasts by cutting them three-quarters of the way through with a sharp knife along one long side. Butterfly them by opening them out like wings and flatten under a piece of clingfilm with a meat tenderizer or base of a small pan. The chicken should be an even thickness to ensure the same cooking time all over.

Season the chicken breasts and rub a little oil over each one.

Grill the breasts until they are cooked through – this will take about 4 minutes each side if the breasts are 2cm (¾in) thick. If you have a meat thermometer, check that the chicken is 80°C (176°F) inside, or cut into the deepest part with a sharp knife to check that the juices run clear and are not pink. The chicken is also delicious barbecued.

Arrange the rocket leaves and Parmesan shavings on a plate or large wooden chopping board. When the chicken is cooked, slice it into strips and transfer to the serving plate. Drizzle the dressing over and serve straight away.

SERVES 4

4 boneless chicken breasts, skinned
1 tablespoon extra virgin olive oil
200g (7oz) rocket leaves or watercress
25g (1oz) Parmesan or Grana Padano, in shavings
salt and freshly ground black pepper

For the dressing

20cm (8in) sprig of rosemary (leaves picked)
½ fresh red chilli (according to taste)
1 small garlic clove
3 tablespoons extra virgin olive oil
1 tablespoon balsamic vinegar

Per serving 0.9g carbs, 35g protein, 16g fat, 1.1g fibre, 292kcal

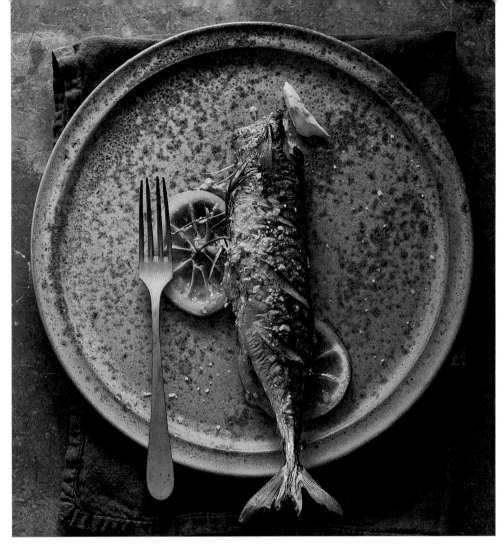

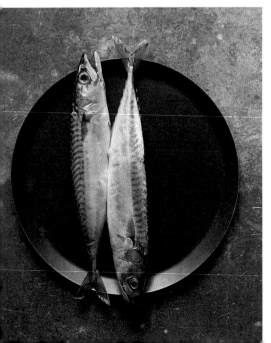

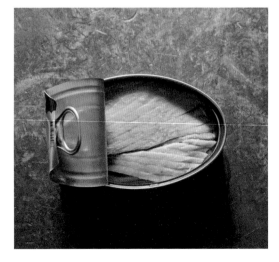

FISH *and* SEAFOOD

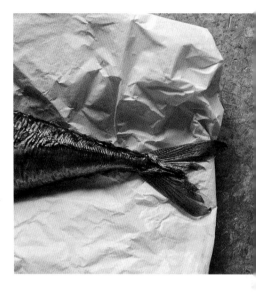

"We don't eat enough fish: can you give us some easy ideas?" seems to be the most frequently asked question at our cookery school. I also hear that many people are worried about cooking fish; that they will overcook it; that it is very expensive; that their partner doesn't like the smell of fish in the house! Here are some easy recipes that serve as a quick lunch or more elaborate dinner to inspire you. Instead of the usual chips, mash and rice as accompaniments, we show you how to serve delicious fish without the carbs.

Oily fish has been eschewed for too long by those on low-fat diets. Here we embrace them as they are full of healthy fats and vitamins, are economical and will fill you up. What's not to like? Nutritionally, there is no difference between fresh and canned fish, so stock up on canned sustainably-caught sardines, pilchards, tuna and mackerel for meals to make in minutes.

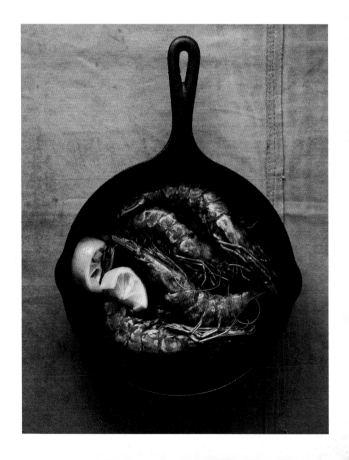

Quick Smoked Mackerel Pâté

This is one of the first recipes I learned in Home Economics lessons at school in the seventies. It is pretty hard to mess up and I remember all of us going home delighted to show our parents what we had made. I've been making it ever since. Serve it on brown bread with any of the breads from Chapter 2, Scandi Seeded Crackers (page 68), lettuce or celery. It keeps well in the fridge for up to 3 days, travels happily and is filling due to the healthy fats in the fish.

Use a fork to mash the cheese together with the remaining ingredients, except the salt and mackerel.

Peel the skin away from the fish and discard. Break up the fish with a fork and stir through the pâté so the finished texture is rough and ready. Season to taste.

Serve with a lemon wedge per person, a scattering of parsley over the top and the Quick Pickled Cucumber on page 152.

SERVES 6

150g (5oz) cream cheese
200g (7oz) full-fat Greek yogurt
juice and zest of 1 lemon
1 teaspoon Dijon mustard, Tabasco, chilli or horseradish sauce
4 tablespoons extra virgin olive oil
1 small garlic clove, very finely chopped
15g (½oz) finely chopped parsley or dill, thick stalks discarded
400g (14oz) smoked peppered mackerel
salt
6 lemon wedges, to serve
small bunch parsley, finely chopped, to serve

Per serving *2.9g carbs, 19g protein, 29g fat, 0g fibre, 350kcal*

Tuna Mayo

I remember when I was a nanny in Long Island, the family I worked for frequently made up batches of this. Now my family love it on lettuce leaves. It will keep in the fridge for a couple of days and it is ideal to take to work. The same recipe works for canned sardines, mackerel or pilchards, too.

Mix all the ingredients together in a bowl and season to taste. Serve on lettuce leaves or low-carb bread (page 69).

SERVES 4

1 x 200g can of tuna, drained
3 tablespoons mayonnaise
3 tablespoons full-fat Greek yogurt
1 celery stick, finely chopped
salt and freshly ground black pepper

Per serving *2.1g carbs, 10g protein, 19g fat, 0g fibre, 218kcal*

SMÖRGÅSBORD

This is an assembly meal that you can throw together in minutes. Fill a chopping board with a selection of peppered smoked mackerel, smoked salmon, smoked trout, hot-smoked salmon, cooked prawns, salmon caviar and lemon wedges. Our son Giorgio makes Quick Pickled Cucumber (page 152) and then we fill bowls with butter or cream cheese, boiled eggs, radishes, celery sticks and gherkins. The Lemon Yogurt Sauce (page 100), Tuna Mayo (see above) or Quick Smoked Mackerel Pâté (see above) are also good. We love the Scandi Seeded Crackers (page 68), breads (pages 66–81) or lettuce leaves for spooning up the fish.

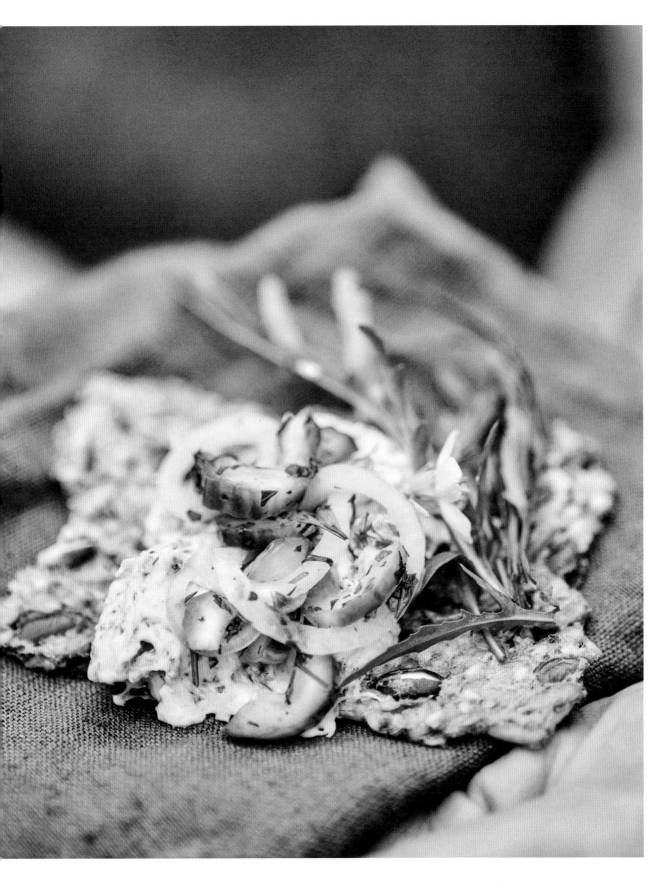

Greek Baked Fish with Tomato Sauce & Onions

Inspired by my travels in Greece, I love the simplicity in this dish and the nutty spice of cinnamon in the sauce. Serve it with salad or the Buttered Medley of Green Vegetables (page 179).

Heat the oil in a heavy-based frying pan. Add the onions, leek, garlic, salt and a good pinch of pepper and fry over a medium heat for 15 minutes, or until the onions and leek have softened.

Add the wine and allow it to reduce for 2 minutes over a high heat. Add the tomatoes, cinnamon, oregano and most of the parsley (reserving 1 tablespoon of the leaves for the end), stir through and bring to the boil. Reduce the heat to low and simmer for 15 minutes.

Meanwhile, preheat the oven to 200°C/fan 180°C/gas mark 6.

Spoon a third of the tomato sauce into a large ovenproof dish. Season the fish and lay the fillets down onto the sauce. Pour the remaining sauce over the top and bake for 15–20 minutes or until the fish is opaque all the way through and breaks apart easily. Serve scattered with the remaining parsley.

SERVES 4

4 tablespoons extra virgin olive oil
3 white onions, finely sliced in half and then from root to tip
1 medium leek, finely sliced
3 garlic cloves, lightly crushed
2 teaspoons salt
100ml (3½fl oz) dry white wine
2 x 400g (14oz) cans of whole plum tomatoes
¼ teaspoon ground cinnamon
2 teaspoons dried oregano
25g (1oz) parsley, leaves roughly chopped and stalks finely chopped
600g (1lb 5oz) halibut or similar white fish fillets, skinned
freshly ground black pepper

Per serving 18g carbs, 4.1g protein, 13g fat, 5g fibre, 241kcal

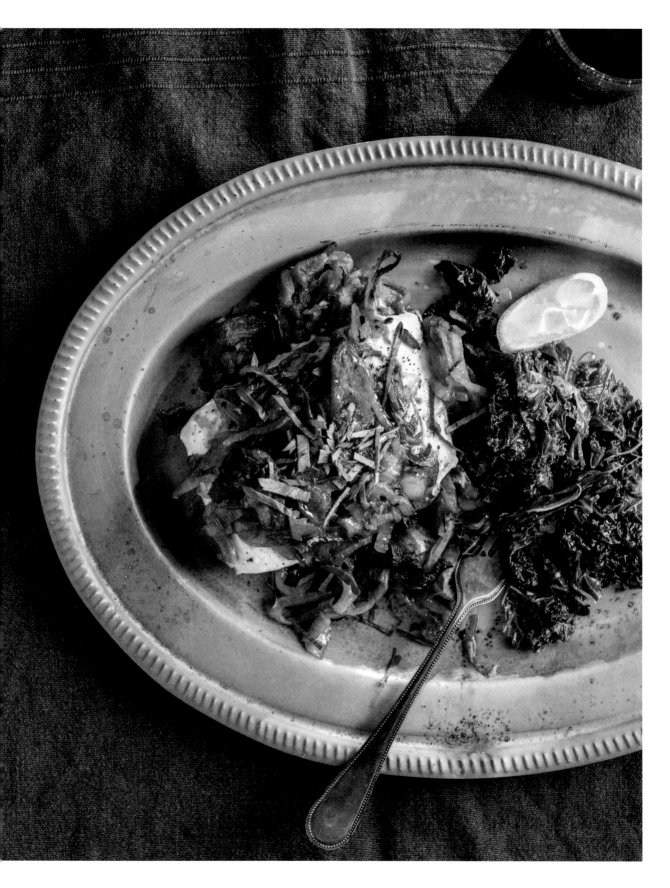

Super Quick Asian Salmon

This is a ridiculously quick and easy dish to throw together and our children love it. It is delicious, healthy food on the table within 15 minutes, so everyone is happy!

Preheat the oven to 200°C/fan 180°C/gas mark 6. Put a large rectangular sheet of baking parchment big enough to hold the fish onto an ovenproof dish. The paper should protrude to catch the liquid.

Lay the salmon on top of the baking parchment. Put all the remaining ingredients on top and spread them out over the fish. Bring the long edges of the parchment together up and over the fish and fold them over several times, leaving a hand-sized gap between the fish and the paper. Twist the ends of the parcel like a sweet to seal in the juices.

Bake for 15–20 minutes until the salmon is firm to the touch and cooked through. Serve on Southeast Asian Cauliflower Rice (page 167) with the juices from the parcel poured over the top, or Southeast Asian Salad (page 153).

SERVES 4

800g (1lb 14oz) salmon, halibut or cod fillet
4 tablespoons tamari
1 stick of lemon grass, finely chopped
1 fat garlic clove, finely sliced
a pinch of chilli flakes or 1 small red chilli (according to taste), sliced (optional)
1 large spring onion, including the green parts, finely sliced
30g (1oz) fresh ginger, peeled and finely chopped
3 tablespoons dry white wine

Per serving 2g carbs, 47g protein, 25g fat, 0g fibre, 444kcal

2-minute Salmon

Split the recipe into individual portions of salmon and topping and use microwave steaming bags – it will cook in about 2 minutes. I used this method when the boys were little and starving hungry, serving it with microwave-steamed broccoli doused in a little toasted sesame oil.

Monkfish à l'Americaine

We were introduced to this heavenly blend of spicy sauce, monkfish and cream by our son Flavio who loves to experiment in the kitchen. The recipe's Breton origin is due to a French chef, Pierre Fraisse, who had worked for a while in Chicago in 1860. He invented the dish, inspired by his travels and named it Sauce Americaine. It can be made with prawns or lobster, too. If your fishmonger gives you the bone, fry it at the same time as the fish to add flavour. The Green Stir-fry on page 172 goes perfectly with this dish.

Season the monkfish on both sides. Heat half the oil in a large frying pan and fry the monkfish (and bone if you have it) for 3 minutes on each side. If water comes out of the fish, don't discard it. Pour in the cognac and leave it to bubble and reduce for 3 minutes.

Meanwhile, fry the shallots and garlic in the remaining oil in another frying pan for 5 minutes.

Add the juices from the monkfish, and the bone if you have it, to the shallots, along with the tomato purée, cayenne pepper and white wine. Bring to the boil, reduce the heat and simmer for 5 minutes before adding the passata. Stir through and let the sauce bubble away gently for 15 minutes.

Add the monkfish and cream and stir through and continue to cook for 10 minutes before serving with the fish.

SERVES 6

1kg (2¼lb) monkfish, off the bone, cut into 5cm (2in) pieces
4 tablespoons extra virgin olive oil
3 tablespoons cognac or brandy
2 shallots, finely chopped
1 garlic clove, finely chopped
2 tablespoons tomato purée
¼ teaspoon cayenne pepper
200ml (7fl oz) dry white wine
1 x 400g (14oz) can of Italian passata
100ml (3½fl oz) double cream
salt and freshly ground black pepper

Per serving 5.4g carbs, 40g protein, 18g fat, 1.6g fibre, 376kcal

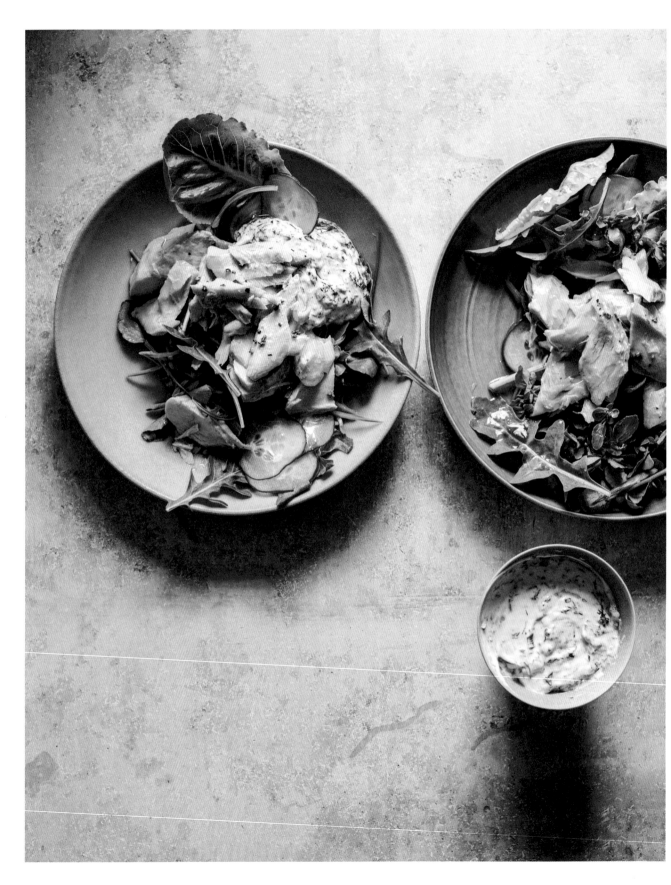

Salmon in a Parcel with Herb Yogurt Sauce

This easy recipe is from Jen Unwin's mother Hazel who whizzes it up quickly in the summer from the herbs she has in her garden. If you only have two or three of the herbs, add more of those to make up the weight. It will still be a lovely sauce and goes well with salad, hot or cold chicken or other oily fish.

Preheat the oven to 200°C/fan180°C/gas mark 6. Cut a piece of baking parchment big enough to overlap a baking tray by 5cm (2in) on each short side. Lay the parchment on top of an equal-sized piece of foil on a baking tray.

Season the salmon on both sides. Lay the fish on the parchment. Scatter the thyme sprigs over the top and drizzle over the wine. Put another piece of parchment on top of the fish and fold the edges together several times, leaving a hand-sized gap between the fish and the paper. This will form a parcel. Do the same with the foil so there is a double layer all around the fish to seal in the juices and steam. Bake for 15–20 minutes until the fish feels firm to the touch.

Meanwhile, make the sauce by whizzing the herbs, oil, lemon juice and seasoning together in a small food-processor. Alternatively, chop the herbs finely by hand. Combine with the yogurt, adjust the seasoning to taste and pour into a serving jug. Store in the fridge until serving; it will keep for up to 4 days.

Serve the salmon on a long plate or wooden board with a jug of the sauce on the side. Mix the lemon juice and oil together and toss with the watercress and some seasoning. Serve the salad by the side of the salmon.

SERVES 6

1kg (2¼lb) salmon fillet
few sprigs of thyme
100ml (3½fl oz) white wine
1 tablespoon lemon juice
2 tablespoons extra virgin olive oil
200g (7oz) watercress
salt and freshly ground black pepper

For the sauce

50g (2oz) mixed herbs, such as mint, dill, chives, parsley, chervil, celery leaves
4 tablespoons extra virgin olive oil
2 tablespoons lemon juice
½ teaspoon salt
½ teaspoon freshly ground black pepper
300g (10½oz) full-fat Greek yogurt

Per serving with sauce

2.9g carbs, 42g protein, 39g fat, 1.4g fibre, 548kcal

Prawn, Chicken & Chorizo Paella

We are delighted with this stunning version of a traditional paella inspired by our friend Nigel Bromilow. He used the traditional paella rice in his version but, with a few adjustments, we have captured all the spicy, saffron-scented flavour without the carbs. I have even served it to friends and they haven't realized it wasn't rice they were tucking into! This makes a big amount for a dinner party, so do choose a large pan.

Heat 1 tablespoon of the oil in a paella dish or large, heavy-based saucepan with a lid. Season the chicken thighs all over and fry, skin side down over a medium-high heat until a rich golden brown. Turn over and continue to fry until browned on all sides. This will take about 25–30 minutes.

Add the chorizo and lardons and fry until crisp. Add two garlic cloves, the onion, red pepper, thyme and chilli flakes and cook until softened.

Pour in the wine and allow to reduce for 5 minutes until the strong smell of alcohol has gone. By this time the chicken should be cooked through. If you have a meat thermometer, check that the chicken is 80°C (176°F) inside, or cut into the deepest part with a sharp knife to check that the juices run clear and are not pink.

Add the cauliflower rice and stir through to combine. Pour in the stock and the saffron and cook for 5 minutes with the lid on. Add the tomatoes and stir through. Continue to cook for a further 4 minutes until the cauliflower is soft.

Meanwhile, heat the remaining oil and garlic in a separate pan and add the prawns. Fry quickly for a couple of minutes until they are pink all over and then add them to the paella. Do the same with the squid, using the garlic oil left in the pan, just until they become opaque and then add them to the paella.

Scatter the parsley over the paella and serve immediately.

SERVES 12

3 tablespoons extra virgin olive oil
8 chicken thighs, skin on, boned and each cut in half
240g (8¾oz) chorizo, cut into thin slices
180g (6½oz) lardons
4 garlic cloves, lightly crushed
2 medium white onions, finely diced
1 red pepper, cut into 1cm-wide strips
1 teaspoon thyme leaves
¼ teaspoon chilli flakes (according to taste)
125ml (4fl oz) dry white wine
1 large cauliflower (approx. 800g/1lb 12oz), riced (page 166)
200ml (7fl oz) hot Chicken Stock (page 115)
1 teaspoon saffron threads, put into stock (above)
4 large tomatoes, deseeded and diced
12 jumbo raw prawns, in shells
450g (1lb) squid, cleaned and chopped into bite-sized pieces
5 tablespoons chopped flat-leaf parsley
salt and freshly ground black pepper

Per serving 9.8g carbs, 32g protein, 21g fat, 2.9g fibre, 437kcal

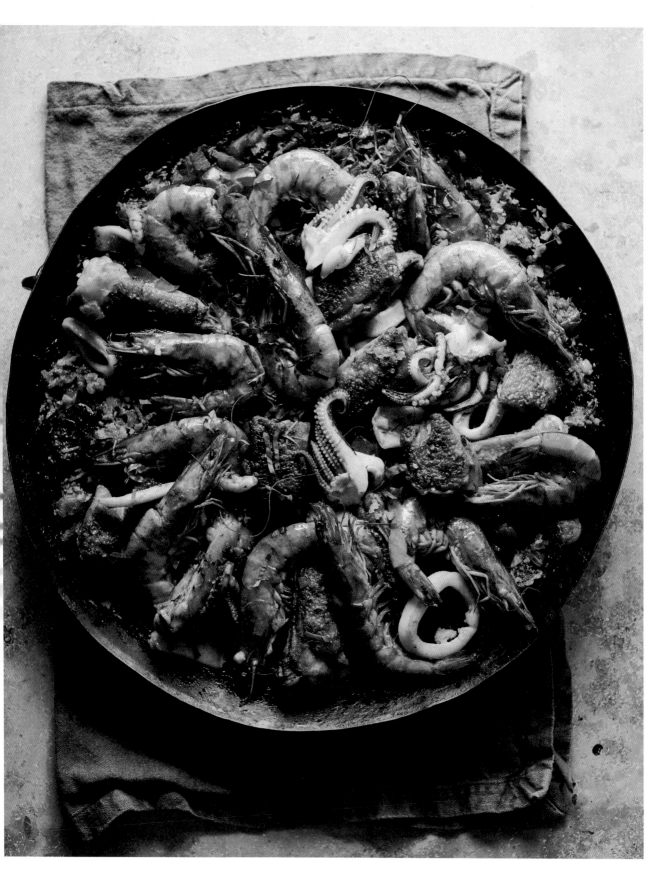

St Lucian Fish Parcel with Green Seasoning

I discovered this wonderful recipe packed with Caribbean colour and flavour while staying in St Lucia at the Cap Maison. Head Chef Craig Jones gave me his recipe and I had a local cooking lesson with the wonderful Matilda, a great grandmother and cook at the Little Lucian Cookery School. She showed me her recipe for the same dish using "green seasoning" – a Caribbean flavour base and marinade for chicken, meat, fish or vegetables before barbecuing or stewing in a clay pot. Try it stirred into any of the Cauliflower Rice recipes on pages 166–167 or the Courgette Ribbons with Avocado & Green Seasoning on page 89.

Serve this with Butternut Squash Curry (page 159) or the Mango & Avocado Salad (page 119).

To make the green seasoning, whizz the ingredients briefly in a food processor to make a rough paste or finely chop them by hand. Use straight away or keep in a jar the fridge for 5 days.

Rub the curry powder and a little salt over the fish on all sides. Put the fish and the green seasoning into a container and stir through. Cover and leave in the fridge for the flavours to infuse for 30 minutes.

Preheat the oven to 200°C/fan180°C/gas mark 6. Place the fish onto a baking tray and drizzle with the oil.

Bake for 12 minutes for flat fish or up to 20 minutes for a fish up to 5cm thick. Remove from the oven and look at the thickest part of the fish to check it is opaque throughout. Serve on a warm platter scattered with the coriander leaves and tomatoes.

SERVES 6

2 teaspoons mild curry powder
900g (2lb) filleted (in one piece) cod or halibut or sea bream, sea bass or red snapper fillets
2 tablespoons melted coconut oil or extra virgin olive oil
salt
a small handful of coriander leaves
6 cherry tomatoes, quartered

For the green seasoning

2 spring onions, including the green parts, or 1 shallot, roughly chopped
1 small green or yellow pepper, roughly chopped
a little finely chopped Scotch bonnet or other hot chilli (according to taste)
20g (¾oz) coriander or flat-leaf parsley, roughly chopped
1 tablespoon thyme leaves
1 garlic clove, peeled
juice of 1 lime
2 tablespoons cold water
½ teaspoon salt

Per serving 0.6g carbs, 36g protein, 7.7g fat, 0g fibre, 215kcal

Fishcakes

These sweet and salty fishcakes take minutes to put together and can be fried or oven baked. Dip into mayonnaise or Lemon Yogurt Sauce (page 104). Alternatively, have them with the Chips (page 171) and a green salad.

If you are cooking the fishcakes in the oven, rather than frying them, preheat the oven to 200°C/fan 180°C/gas mark 6.

Mash the sweet potato to a thick paste in a mixing bowl with a fork. Drain the fish and discard the oil. Add the fish and the remaining ingredients to the bowl except the oil for frying and mash again with a fork until well combined. Season to taste with salt and pepper.

Divide the mixture into four or 8 and use your hands to shape it into flattened patties about 2cm deep. Fry in a little oil in a non-stick frying pan for about 5 minutes each side or until browned and cooked through. Alternatively, oven bake for 20 minutes or until cooked through.

SERVES 2/MAKES 8 small fishcakes or 4 large fishcakes

75g (2¾oz) sweet potato, baked or microwaved and peeled
2 x 120g (4¼oz) cans of mackerel, sardines or pilchards in olive oil
3 spring onions, very finely chopped
15g (½oz) parsley or dill, finely chopped
1 egg
finely grated zest of 1 lemon
extra virgin olive oil, for frying
salt and freshly ground black pepper

Per serving 11g carbs, 31g protein, 26g fat, 2.1g fibre, 402kcal

Fish Pie

By swapping potato for celeriac here we have cut the carbs and have enriched the dish with cream and eggs. You can use any inexpensive white fish, such as coley, or use fish trimmings. Salmon or prawns make it pretty and don't forget to include a little smoked fish for flavour. Swap the celeriac mash for cauliflower mash, if you prefer.

Preheat the oven to 200°C/fan 180°C/gas mark 6.

Boil the celeriac in plenty of salted water for about 10 minutes, or until tender when pierced with a knife. Drain and blitz in a food-processor or with a stick blender with 50g (2oz) of the butter until smooth. Season to taste and set aside.

To make the béchamel, follow the method on page 100.

Put the fish and sliced boiled eggs into a lasagne dish measuring 22 x 28cm (8½ x 11in) and scatter over a little salt and pepper. Pour over the béchamel and use a fork to make sure the pieces of fish and egg are covered. Use a tablespoon to dollop on the mash in little heaps over the surface and then join them together. Make lines over the surface with the tines of a fork. Dot with the remaining butter and bake for 35–40 minutes or until golden brown. Serve.

SERVES 6

800g (1lb 12oz) celeriac, peeled and roughly chopped
70g (2½oz) butter
1 quantity Béchamel (page 100)
800g (1lb 14oz) mixed fish fillets, cut into bite-sized pieces
4 boiled eggs, cooled, peeled and thickly sliced
salt and freshly ground black pepper

Per serving 3.2g carbs, 39g protein, 18g fat, 5g fibre, 344kcal

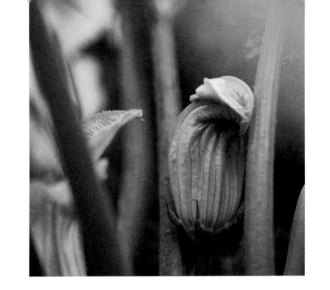

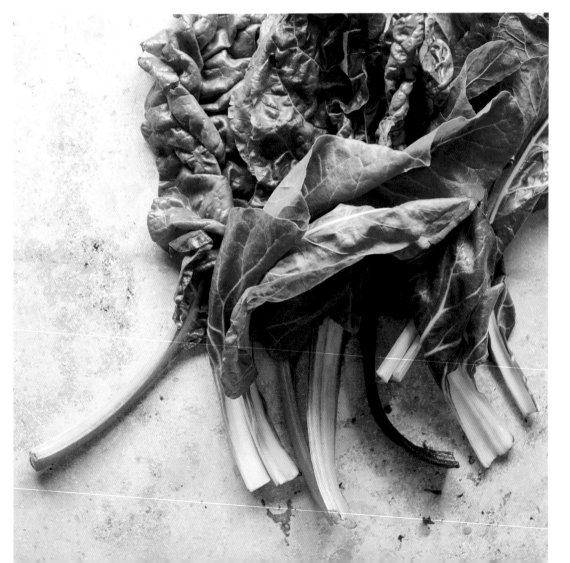

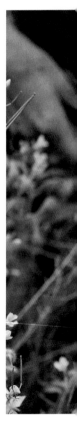

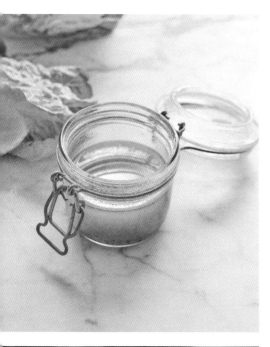

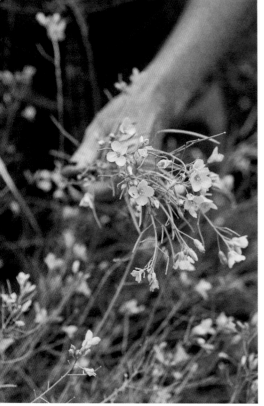

VEGETABLES

There are rising numbers of people following a vegetarian or vegan diet. Whatever your reason for being meat-free, it is important to make sure you consume enough protein and healthy fats to be satiated, otherwise you will be reaching for the biscuit tin again and again. For this reason, we have suggested some additional and optional sources of vegetarian protein, such as lentils, farro or chickpeas. Each of these contains carbs though, so go easy if you are low on the CarbScale (page 21).

Adding butter or olive oil, together with a sprinkling of salt and pepper, makes vegetables extremely tasty and it also helps your body to absorb the fat-soluble vitamins, such as vitamins K and A. We're sure more children and adults would eat their greens if they were served this way.

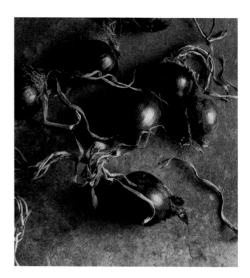

Roasted Vegetable Soup with Mint & Goat's Cheese

We love this hearty, comforting soup full of the flavours of the Mediterranean. By using a low-carb vegetable such as swede you can achieve a dense soup without using potato or flour. While the soup cooks you can roast the vegetables.

Preheat the oven to 220°C/fan 200°C/gas mark 7.

For the tomato base, heat the oil in a large saucepan. Sauté the base vegetables with the thyme for about 10 minutes until they begin to stick to the base of the pan. Add the canned tomatoes, along with the basil, followed by the hot stock or water. Bring to the boil and then reduce the heat and simmer, with a lid on ajar, until the vegetables are soft. This will take 20–30 minutes.

Meanwhile, put the roasting vegetables onto an oven tray and toss in the oil and seasoning. Spread them out in a single layer with the rosemary tucked underneath and roast for 20–25 minutes, or until they are tender.

Purée the tomato base with a stick blender or in a food-processor. Return the soup to the pan. Stir in the spinach and taste for seasoning. Divide into warm bowls and top with the mint, roasted vegetables, spoonfuls of goat's cheese and the seeds.

SERVES 4

For the tomato base
3 tablespoons extra virgin olive oil
1 leek, roughly chopped
2 celery sticks, roughly chopped
300g (10½oz) swede, peeled and roughly chopped
2 sprigs of thyme
2 x 400g (14oz) cans of Italian plum tomatoes
1 sprig of basil
1 litre (1¾ pints) hot vegetable stock, Chicken Stock (page 115) or hot water

For the roasted vegetables
1 red pepper, cut into 2cm (¾in)pieces
1 medium aubergine, diced into 2cm (¾in) cubes
1 red onion, cut into 2cm (¾in) cubes
1 courgette, roughly chopped into 2cm (¾in) slices
2 sprigs rosemary
4 tablespoons extra virgin olive oil
salt and freshly ground black pepper

To finish
250g (9oz) baby spinach
a large handful of mint leaves, roughly torn
150g (5oz) soft goat's cheese
2 tablespoons toasted pumpkin or mixed seeds

Per serving 22g carbs, 16g protein, 36g fat, 8.9g fibre, 496kcal

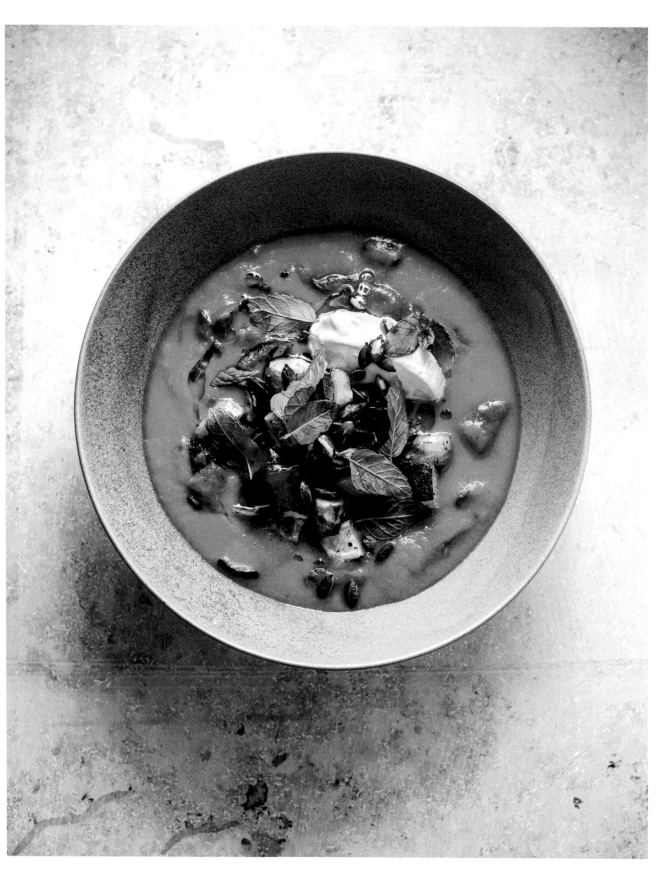

Broccoli, Eggs & Tahini Sauce

The creamy, nutty dressing brings out the best in a simple boiled egg and makes the perfect dipping sauce for broccoli spears. It also marries well with roasted vegetables and salads.

Lower the eggs into a pan of boiling water and cook for 8 minutes. Meanwhile, steam or boil the broccoli for 3–4 minutes with a little salt until tender. Drain and drizzle with a little oil and season with salt and pepper. Keep warm until serving.

Once the eggs are cooked, drain and plunge them into cold water. Crack the shells straight away to prevent a ring of blue forming around the yolks. Cut each one in half after peeling.

To make the dressing, put all the ingredients in a small bowl or jar. Add 3 tablespoons of cold water (double this if making a runny dressing), mix well and season to taste. Use straight away or keep in the fridge for up to 3 days.

Spoon the tahini sauce into little bowls and sit them on 4 plates with the eggs, broccoli and pepper strips ready to be dipped. Scatter with coriander and serve.

SERVES 4/MAKES 100ml (3½fl oz) dressing

8 large eggs
250g (9oz) Tenderstem broccoli spears
extra virgin olive oil, for drizzling
1 red pepper, cut into 1cm (½in) strips
a small handful of coriander, roughly chopped
salt and freshly ground black pepper

For the tahini sauce
3 tablespoons tahini
2 tablespoons extra virgin olive oil
1 medium garlic clove, finely grated
2 tablespoons lemon juice, plus extra to taste

Per serving 3.3g carbs, 21g protein, 29g fat, 3.4g fibre, 363 kcal

Italian Roasted Vegetables

We probably make these three times a week at home – we love the flavour that roasted onion, herbs and garlic bring to the humble vegetable. Always tuck the herbs under the vegetables to give flavour and stop them burning, and space the vegetables out so that they roast rather than steam in a pile.

Preheat the oven to 220°C/fan 200°C/gas mark 7. Grease a baking tray with a little of the oil.
Put the vegetables and rosemary into a bowl with the remaining oil and season with a large pinch of salt and pepper. Toss to combine. Spread the vegetables over the tray evenly in one layer (you may have to use two trays).

Roast for 30 minutes until cooked through and golden brown on top. Serve.

SERVES 2 for a main course or 4 as a side

4 tablespoons extra virgin olive oil
1 aubergine, sliced lengthways into 1cm (½in) thick strips
1 courgette, cut into 1cm (½in) slices
1 red or yellow pepper, cut into finger-width strips
1 onion, cut into finger-width wedges
2 garlic cloves, lightly crushed
2 sprigs of rosemary
salt and freshly ground black pepper

Per serving (as a side) 7.1g carbs, 2.2g protein, 13g fat, 4g fibre, 162kcal

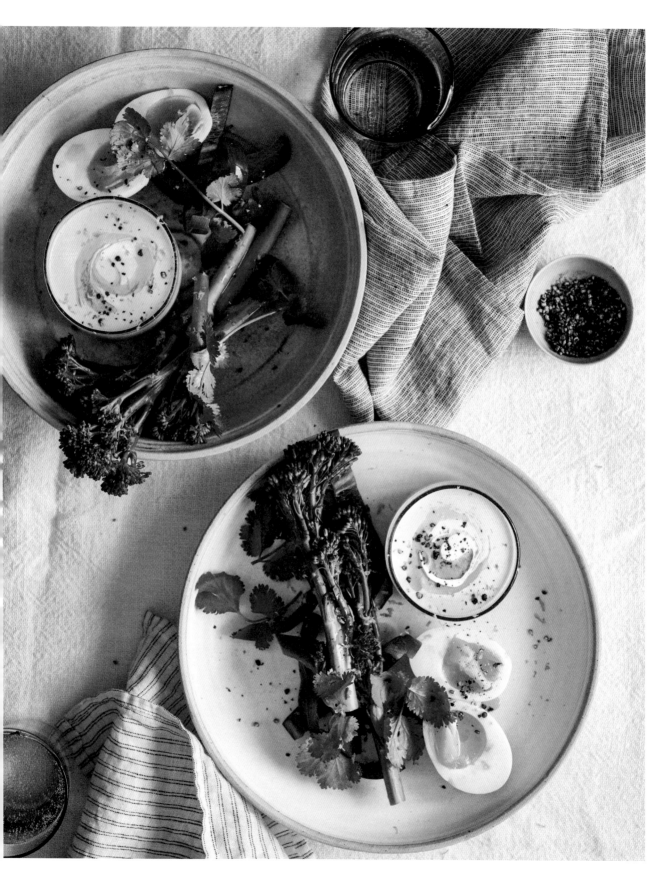

Smoked Cheese, Leek & Cauliflower Soup

This quick and simple soup uses up ends of cheese leftover in the fridge. We love smoked Cheddar, but any cheese that melts easily will work.

We finely slice the inside of the green end of a leek for the topping, but other ideas are endless: leftover roast vegetables, roast cherry tomatoes, crumbled feta cheese, fried cubes of halloumi… The cream, almonds and seeds add nutrients and will keep you fuller for longer. You can use broccoli instead of cauliflower and speed up the process by leaving out the topping if all you are interested in is a bowl of comfort.

Heat half the fat in a large, heavy-based saucepan. Add the leeks and thyme and sauté for 5 minutes. Add the cauliflower and stock or water and bring to the boil. Continue to boil gently for a few minutes or until the cauliflower is tender. Remove the thyme sprigs and purée the soup with a stick blender or liquidizer to a smooth consistency, taking care the hot soup doesn't splash you.

Add the cream and cheese and stir over the heat until the cheese has melted. Season to taste. Keep the soup warm while you prepare the topping.

Fry the cauliflower leaves and stalks, leek trimmings and garlic in the remaining fat for about 3 minutes. Add the flaked almonds and seeds and stir through. Season to taste.

Serve the soup into warm bowls with the topping divided between them.

SERVES 6

2 tablespoons ghee, butter or chicken fat
2 medium leeks (250g/9oz after trimming), roughly chopped (keep the ends for later)
2 sprigs of thyme
550g (1¼lb) cauliflower, cut into small florets
1 litre (1¾ pints) vegetable stock, Chicken Stock (page 115) or hot water
100ml (3½fl oz) double cream
50g (2oz) smoked or other cheese, finely grated
salt and freshly ground black pepper

For the topping
100g (3½oz) cauliflower leaves and stalks, very finely sliced
trimmings from the end of 1 leek (see above) or 2 spring onions, finely sliced
2 garlic cloves, finely chopped
50g (2oz) flaked almonds
2 tablespoons sunflower seeds
extra virgin olive oil

Per serving *13g carbs, 8.2g protein, 24g fat, 5.3g fibre, 306kcal*

ROAST CAULIFLOWER LEAVES & STEMS
Cast out into the darkness of the bin, these unloved parts of a cauliflower are now stepping out into the limelight. Enjoy them with a little butter or splash over a little soy sauce, toasted sesame oil and sesame seeds before putting in the oven.

Preheat the oven to 220°C/fan 200°C/gas mark 7. Rub a little olive oil and seasoning into the leaves and stems and spread them out on a baking tray. Roast for 5–7 minutes or until the leaves become translucent and crisp. Serve warm. If you remove the stems from the leaves the stems can be cooked as chips (see page 171). The leaves on their own prepared in this way will only take 3–4 minutes to crisp up.

Mushroom & Tahini Soup

I discovered this soup on a fascinating trip to Thessaloniki in northern Greece. Tahini helps to thicken the soup as well as impart its rich, earthy flavour. My teacher Sakis Kalliontzis makes it with seasonal mushrooms throughout the year.

Heat the oil and butter together in a large saucepan. Once bubbling, sauté the mushrooms, garlic, thyme and other vegetables for 10 minutes, then add the water or stock. Bring to the boil, reduce the heat and simmer for 30 minutes or until all the vegetables are tender.

Meanwhile, to finish, heat the oil in a frying pan and sauté the mushrooms, garlic and thyme until lightly browned. Discard the garlic and thyme, set aside the mushrooms and keep warm.

Remove the thyme sprigs from the large saucepan and purée the mushrooms and vegetables with a stick blender or liquidizer to a smooth consistency, taking care the hot soup doesn't splash you.

Add the tahini and cream (if using) and blend again. Taste and add more tahini if you like it.

Heat the soup once more in the pan, before serving in warm bowls scattered with the sautéed mushrooms, parsley and pistachios.

SERVES 8

2 tablespoons extra virgin olive oil
50g (2oz) butter
500g (18oz) chestnut or button
  mushrooms, peeled and halved
2 garlic cloves, lightly crushed
few sprigs of thyme
1 medium leek, finely sliced
1 carrot, roughly chopped
200g (7oz) celeriac, peeled and
  roughly chopped or 2 celery sticks,
  roughly chopped
1.5 litres (2¾ pints) hot water,
  vegetable stock or Chicken Stock
  (page 115)
2–3 tablespoons tahini, to taste
5 tablespoons double cream
  (optional)

To finish

2 tablespoons extra virgin olive oil
100g (3½oz) mushrooms, brushed
  clean and finely sliced
1 garlic clove, peeled
1 sprig of thyme
a small handful of parsley, stems
  removed, roughly chopped
3 tablespoons pistachios, roughly
  chopped

Per serving *5g carbs, 4.8g protein, 23g fat, 3.1g fibre, 248kcal*

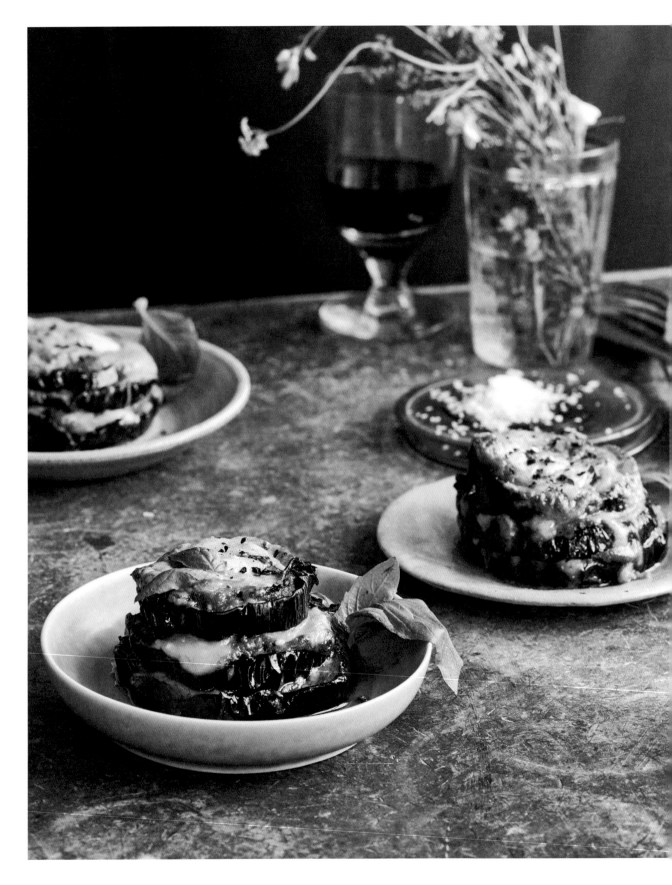

Aubergine Parmigiana

This classic Italian recipe is inherently low-carb, however the aubergines are often coated in flour or breadcrumbs and then deep-fried. We were shown this lighter and simpler version with smoked cheese and roast aubergines in Amalfi. We have given two options for assembly: the towers which look great and are ideal for lunch or a starter for dinner, or a large bake which is perfect for a family supper.

Cut or tear the mozzarella into pieces and drain in a sieve for 1 hour, or up to overnight in the fridge.

Preheat the oven to 220°C/fan 200°C/gas mark 7. Grease a baking tray with a little oil.

Meanwhile, lay the aubergine slices onto the prepared tray. Brush with oil and season lightly with salt and pepper. Roast the aubergines for 25–30 minutes, or until lightly browned. Remove from the oven and leave to cool briefly.

Purée the tomato sauce with a stick blender or in a food-processor until smooth. (See below for how to assemble the towers or bake.)

SERVES 6

2 x 125g (4½oz) balls buffalo mozzarella
extra virgin olive oil, to grease the tray and brush the aubergines
3 aubergines, cut into 1cm (½in) thick slices
1 quantity tomato sauce (page 90)
12 broad basil leaves
25g (1oz) Parmesan, finely grated
25g (1oz) smoked Provola cheese or smoked Cheddar, finely grated
salt and freshly ground black pepper

Per serving *8.1g carbs, 13g protein, 26g fat, 3.6g fibre, 332kcal*

Variations

TO MAKE INDIVIDUAL AUBERGINE TOWERS
Match together similar-sized aubergine circles – you will need three for each tower. Spoon 1 heaped dessertspoon of tomato sauce onto one circle. Top with a basil leaf and a little of each cheese. Add another aubergine circle and repeat with the sauce, leaf and cheese. Top with the final aubergine circle followed by the sauce, leaf and cheese. Repeat for the remaining towers, place in an ovenproof dish and bake for about 45 minutes or until the cheese is lightly browned.

FOR AN AUBERGINE BAKE
Pour one-third of the tomato sauce into a medium lasagne dish and lay over one-third of the aubergine slices. Top with one-third of each cheese and one-third of the basil leaves. Repeat twice more, finishing with the cheese. Bake for 45 minutes–1 hour, or until the cheese is lightly browned.

Leek, Spinach & Feta Showstopper

This is really an assembly of ingredients rather than complicated cooking, yet the result is a spectacular dish topped with an irresistible savoury crumble to impress vegetarian and meat-eating friends alike. To save time, buy frozen spinach and a jar of roasted red peppers.

Preheat the oven to 200°C/fan 180°C/gas mark 6. Generously grease a 20cm (8in) springform cake tin with some butter.

Prepare the leeks first using as much of the green end as you can, unless they are very tough. Cut them finely into half-moons. Put the leeks into a large frying pan with the butter, oil, ¼ teaspoon of salt and some black pepper and fry gently until tender – about 10 minutes.

Leave the leeks to cool and then mix with the ricotta, feta and two of the eggs. Season again to taste.

Squeeze the excess water from the spinach and whizz in a food-processor with the remaining egg, ¼ teaspoon of salt, some black pepper and the nutmeg.

Make the crumble by rubbing the butter into the almonds and Parmesan in a mixing bowl.

Make the base of the cake by opening out the peppers and patting them dry with a kitchen paper. Lay them down to fit the base of the prepared tin, cutting them as necessary. They should come up the side by 1.5cm(⅝in) all around.

Next spoon half the leek mixture into the tin and press down lightly with the back of a spoon. Now do the same with the spinach mixture and then with the last of the leek mix. Sprinkle the crumble over the top in an even layer and place on a baking tray in case of any leaks.

Bake for 30 minutes or until the crumble is golden brown. Leave the crumble to cool for 10 minutes before transferring to a serving dish. Serve warm or at room temperature.

SERVES 10

10g (¼oz) butter, plus extra to grease
500g (18oz) leeks (trimmed weight)
2 tablespoons extra virgin olive oil
250g (9oz) ricotta
100g (3½oz) feta, grated
3 eggs, beaten
900g–1kg (2–2¼lb) frozen spinach, or 300g (10½oz) cooked and squeezed spinach
¼ teaspoon freshly grated nutmeg
200g (7oz) roasted red peppers (drained weight)
salt and freshly ground black pepper

For the crumble
25g (1oz) cold salted butter, diced
100g (3½oz) ground almonds
50g (2oz) Parmesan, finely grated

Per serving 5.2g carbs, 18g protein, 24g fat, 4.6g fibre, 314kcal

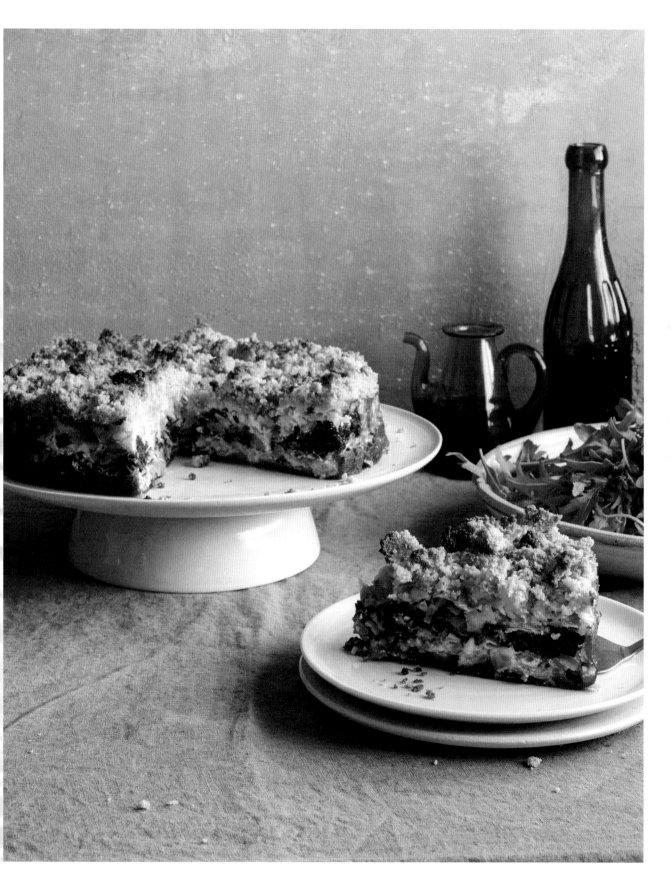

Quick Pickled Cucumber

This crunchy, fresh-tasting salad is the ideal partner for oily fish or with the Quick Smoked Mackerel Pâté (page 128). Use small cucumbers that have fewer seeds, if you can find them.

Cut some of the skin of the cucumbers away lengthways to create long thick or thin stripes. This can be done with a potato peeler.

Cut the cucumbers in half lengthways and use a teaspoon to scrape out the seeds. Next lay the cucumber halves, cut-side down, onto a board and slice into half-moon shapes, about 2mm (1/16in) wide. Mix them in a bowl with the salt and then put into a sieve to drain for 30 minutes.

Gently press the cucumbers into the sieve with a large spoon to rid them of any remaining water. Mix with all the remaining ingredients in a bowl. Season to taste. Toss to combine and serve straight away or store, in a covered container, for up to 3 days in the fridge.

SERVES 6

4 small cucumbers or 1 English long
  cucumber
1 teaspoon salt
1 shallot, thinly sliced
1 tablespoon finely chopped dill
1 tablespoon finely chopped parsley
2 tablespoons cider vinegar

Per serving 1.7g carbs,
1.2g protein, 0.7g fat, 1.1g fibre,
20kcal

Green Salad with Vinaigrette

I always like to throw a handful of herbs, and their flowers when in season, into a salad and I try to use a variety of leaves to get a broad scope of micronutrients. Other addtions could be green pepper, fresh chilli, capers, olives, nuts or toasted seeds. I have been making this dressing ever since my mother taught me when I was about five years old. Now our sons make it, too.

Put all the salad ingredients into a serving bowl.

Put all the vinaigrette ingredients into a jar with a good pinch of pepper and shake well to emulsify.

Dress the salad with the vinaigrette just before serving, gently tossing it with tongs. Keep any remaining dressing in the fridge for up to a week.

**SERVES 6/MAKES approx. 125ml
(4fl oz)**

For the salad
200g (7oz) mixed salad leaves
1/3 cucumber, finely sliced
1 celery stick, finely sliced
a handful of herbs, such as parsley,
  chives, coriander, fresh oregano, basil

For the vinaigrette
1 teaspoon Dijon mustard
2 tablespoons red wine vinegar
8 tablespoons extra virgin olive oil
1/2 teaspoon salt
1 tablespoon lemon juice
1 small garlic clove, grated
freshly ground black pepper

Per serving 1.5g carbs, 1g protein,
17g fat, 0.8g fibre, 169kcal

Southeast Asian Salad

Our family holiday in Vietnam got us hooked on Southeast Asian salads. We love the balance of colour, texture and sweet and sour. My sister, Louli, has experimented with the dressings and has managed to reduce the usual sweetness to just 1 teaspoon of honey.

Soak the spring onions in cold water for 10 minutes to take out their strength. Dry-fry the nuts (if using) in a small frying pan until lightly browned. Remove from the heat, transfer to a plate and leave to cool. Toast the sesame seeds in the same pan for a few minutes over a medium heat until golden. Remove from the heat, transfer to the plate and leave to cool.

Make up the dressing by whisking all the ingredients together in a bowl or shaking in a jar. Season to taste.

Drain the spring onions and mix with the remaining salad ingredients and dressing in a large, shallow bowl or plate. Scatter over the nuts (if using) and seeds and serve.

SERVES 4

3 spring onions, finely chopped
a small handful of peanuts or
  almonds, roughly chopped (optional)
1 tablespoon sesame seeds
200g (7oz) white cabbage, finely
  shredded
1 unripe mango, peeled, stoned and
  finely sliced
1 Romano or red pepper, finely sliced
25g (1oz) coriander, leaves roughly
  chopped and stalks finely chopped
a small handful of mint leaves
100g (3½oz) mangetout, finely sliced
  lengthways

For the dressing
juice of 2 limes
1 garlic clove, finely grated
1 small red chilli, finely chopped,
  added according to taste
2 tablespoons fish sauce
1 teaspoon mild clear honey
  (optional)
salt and freshly ground black pepper

Per serving 12g carbs,
4.9g protein, 4.9g fat, 5g fibre,
125kcal

A Great Greek Salad

This stunning salad is inspired by a recipe from the restaurant Apeirotan Taverna in Thessaloniki. It was served in a huge mound that formed a centrepiece on the table for us all to share. I loved the fact that it wasn't mixed together so you could help yourself to the various flavours and textures. If you have a food-processor this is a very quick salad to prepare with the grater and blade attachments. Vary the vegetables according to the season and what you have in the fridge.

Soak the spring onions in cold water for 10 minutes to take out their strength.

Mix the oil with the lemon juice in a small bowl and season to taste.

Put the carrots and apple into a bowl with a little of the oil and lemon mixture and toss to combine to stop them becoming brown. Put the carrot and apple salad onto an area of a serving board.

Mix the red cabbage with the walnuts, drained onions, dill and a little of the oil and lemon mixture and add to the board. Do the same with the broccoli and lentils (if using). Put the red pepper and seeds straight onto the board. Any remaining oil and lemon mixture can be poured over the salad.

The salad will keep like this in the fridge for a few hours before serving. Serve the tahini dressing in a jug on the side.

SERVES 6

4 spring onions, including the green parts, finely chopped
100ml (3½fl oz) extra virgin olive oil
juice of 1 lemon
3 medium carrots, coarsely grated
1 large apple, cored and coarsely grated or chopped
¼ red cabbage, coarsely grated or finely sliced
30g (1¼oz) walnuts, toasted and roughly chopped
20g (¾oz) dill fronds or roughly chopped parsley
150g (5oz) broccoli, finely chopped
250g (9oz) cooked Puy lentils (optional)
1 red pepper, finely sliced
30g (1¼oz) pumpkin or sunflower seeds, toasted
1 quantity Tahini Sauce (page 144), thinned with 3 tablespoons water
salt and freshly ground black pepper

Tahini dressing per serving
0g carbs, 3g protein, 17g fat, 1.1g fibre, 172kcal
Per serving of salad with lentils
18g carbs, 8.3g protein, 23g fat, 7.2g fibre, 330kcal
Per serving of salad without lentils 12g carbs, 4.7g protein, 23g fat, 5.7g fibre, 285kcal

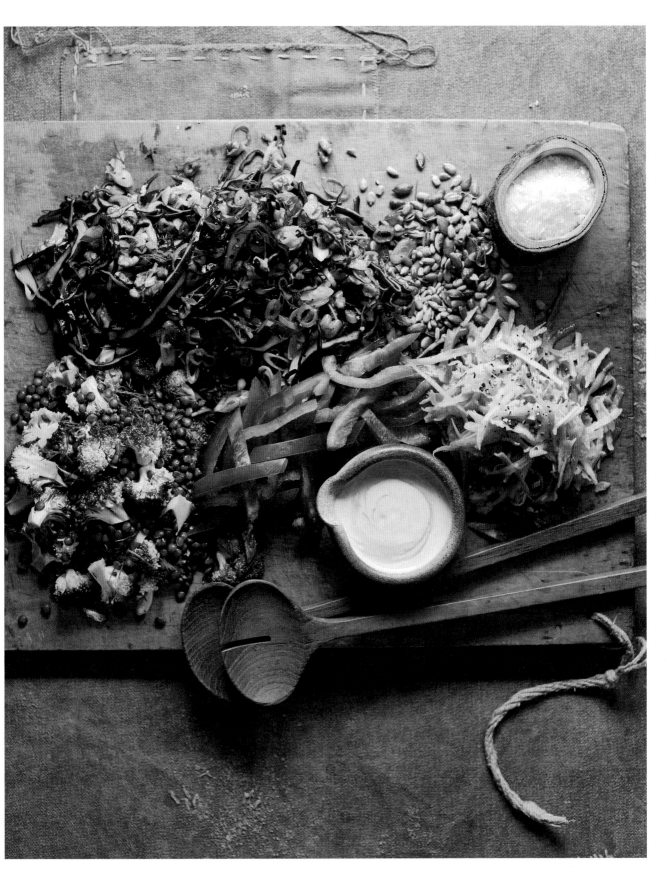

Courgette Fetta, Labneh & Dukkah

"Fetta" means slice and refers to the grilled courgettes in this dish, though it can be made with any vegetable that can be grilled. You can buy labneh (strained yogurt) or use very thick Greek yogurt. Just make sure it contains live bacteria as that is what is so nourishing. Dukkah is an Egyptian coarsely ground mixture of nuts, seeds and spices served with bread dunked in oil. You can buy it ready-made, but below is our friend Amal's recipe.

Preheat the oven to 220°C/fan 200°C/gas mark 7.

Lay the courgettes and tomatoes on a baking tray and wipe over 1 tablespoon of the oil with your fingers. Sprinkle with the cumin and turmeric, and some salt and pepper, and bake for 15 minutes.

Remove from the oven and arrange on a plate. Dress with the labneh, sumac, dukkah, remaining oil and mint leaves and serve.

SERVES 6 as a side or 2 as a main course

4 courgettes, cut into 3 long slices 0.5cm (¼in) thick
2 handfuls of cherry tomatoes, cut in half around their middle
2 tablespoons extra virgin olive oil
1 teaspoon ground cumin
1 teaspoon ground turmeric
100g (3½oz) labneh or thick Greek yogurt
½ teaspoon sumac or paprika
3 tablespoons dukkah
a handful of mint leaves, roughly torn
salt and freshly ground black pepper

Per serving of courgette fetta
4.9g carbs, 4.6g protein, 6.2g fat, 3.4g fibre, 102kcal
Per serving of dukkah 2.1g carbs, 4.2g protein, 14g fat, 1.7g fibre, 151kcal

To make your own dukkah

MAKES approx. 300g (10½oz)/SERVES 12

250g (9oz) mixed nuts, such as hazelnuts, pecans, pine nuts, flaked almonds, pistachios, walnuts
35g (1¼oz) seeds, such as white or black sesame, sunflower, pumpkin
1 tablespoon cumin seeds
1 tablespoon coriander seeds
1 teaspoon sea salt flakes

Preheat the oven to 190°C/fan 170°C/gas mark 5. Line a baking tray with baking parchment.

Stir all the ingredients together in a bowl and then spread them onto the lined tray. Bake for 15–20 minutes or until lightly browned.

Remove from the oven and leave to cool for 10 minutes. Pound the mixture in a pestle and mortar, chop by hand with a sharp knife on a board or whizz briefly in a food-processor until the nuts are broken down and you have the textures of both gravel and sand. Leave to cool completely and then store in a jar until needed. The dukkah will keep for a few weeks at room temperature.

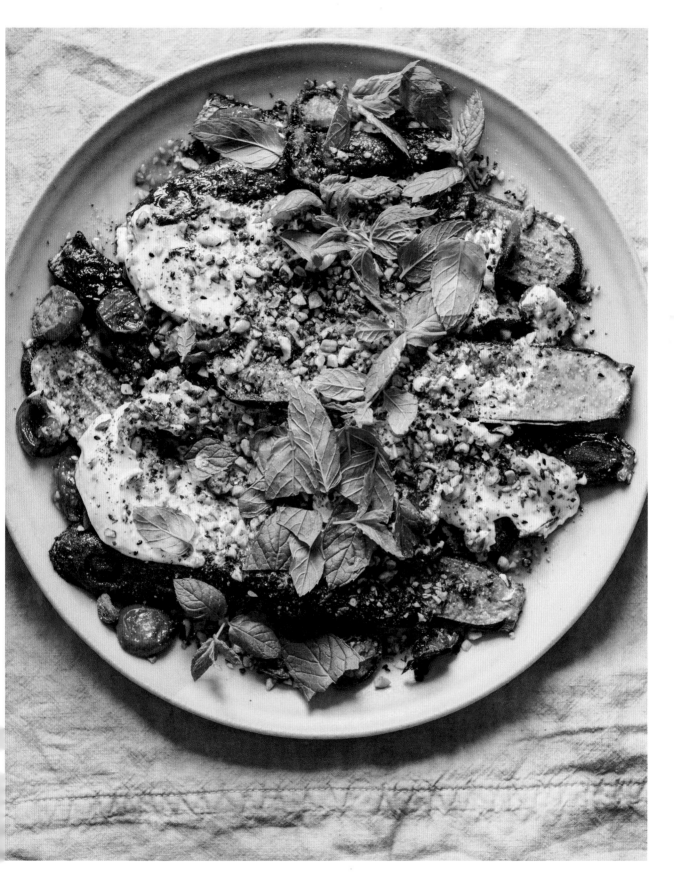

Bouyiourdi

Bouyiourdi is a traditional dish from Thessaloniki – northern Greece's fascinating foodie capital. Bouyiourdi (pronounced "booyoordee") is a wondrous combination of melted cheese, tomatoes, oregano and chilli (see images overleaf). It is sold all over the city in various guises, some made with tomato sauce (page 90) instead of fresh tomatoes and others with roast red peppers. Serve it hot and gooey with chicory leaves, Baguettes (page 72) or a green salad (page 152).

Preheat the oven to 240°C/fan 220°C/gas mark 9.

Lay a third of the tomatoes in the base of a small ovenproof dish. Follow this with a third of the sheep's cheese and the slab of feta. Add another two layers of tomatoes and sheep's cheese, finishing with more tomatoes and the fresh chillies.

Drizzle with the oil and scatter over the chilli flakes and oregano. Seal the baking dish tightly with foil and bake for 20 minutes. Remove the foil and bake for a further 15 minutes. Serve straight away.

SERVES 4

3 large ripe tomatoes (approx. 325g/11oz), diced into 2cm (¾in) cubes or the same weight of tomato sauce (page 90)

100g (3½oz) hard sheep's cheese (saganaki, Manchego, pecorino, Cheddar), roughly cut into 0.5cm (¼in) thick slices

200g (7oz) feta

½ mild red chilli (according to taste), finely sliced

½ mild green chilli (according to taste), finely sliced

1 tablespoon extra virgin olive oil

¼ teaspoon chilli flakes (according to taste)

1 teaspoon dried oregano

Per serving 3.7g carbs, 12g protein, 18g fat, 1g fibre, 233kcal

Butternut Squash Curry

This is a little higher in carbs than most recipes in the book, but you can serve it in small portions. Butternut squash is available all year, but when pumpkin is in season use this as the carbs are lower. This is delicious served with the St Lucian Fish Parcel (page 138).

Make the paste in a food-processor by blitzing the ingredients together with a few twists of black pepper. Alternatively, chop everything finely by hand.

Heat the oil in a medium-sized saucepan. Fry the paste for 5 minutes over a low heat.

Stir the squash into the paste and continue to fry for 3 minutes, then add the coconut milk. Bring to the boil, reduce the heat to low and cook for 30 minutes, or until the squash is soft and tender. Serve.

SERVES 6

2 tablespoons coconut oil or extra virgin olive oil
400g (14oz) butternut squash or pumpkin flesh, cut into 2cm (¾in) cubes
1 x 400g (14oz) can of coconut milk

For the curry paste
1 white onion, roughly chopped
15g (½oz) fresh ginger, peeled and roughly chopped
1 fat garlic clove, peeled
½ orange pepper
small bunch coriander (15g/½oz)
½ teaspoon salt
freshly ground black pepper

Butternut squash per serving
14g carbs, 7g protein, 41g fat, 5.7g fibre, 467kcal

Pumpkin squash per serving
9.7g carbs, 6.8g protein, 41g fat, 3.3g fibre, 445kcal

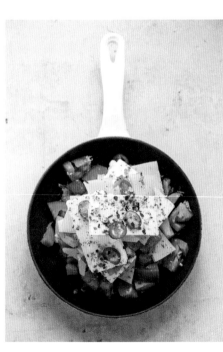
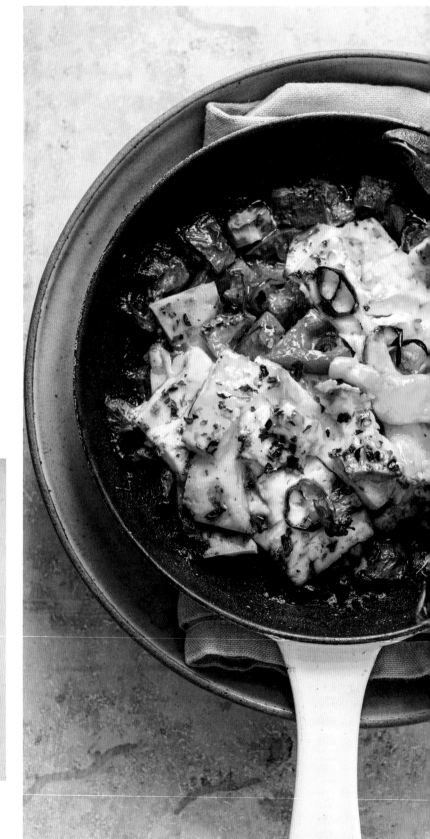

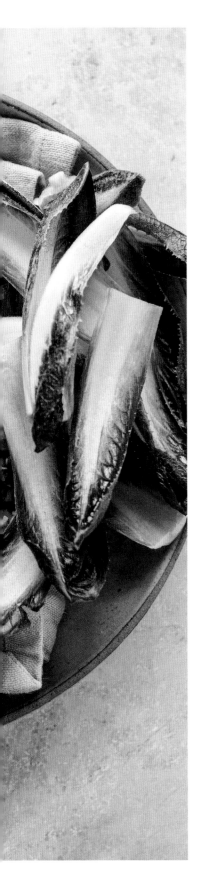

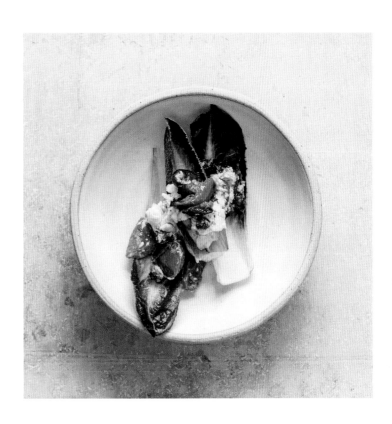

Masala Curry Base

Masala means "mixture" and it refers to the blend of spices used to give a typically Asian flavour to food. This curry base goes perfectly with eggs (see below), vegetables (see opposite) or chickpeas and was shown to us by our friend Sohini Basu when we were in Calcutta together. We all adore this recipe in our family and often cook it to accompany the Spicy Paneer (page 174). It will keep in the fridge for a few days.

Heat the fat in a large saucepan or frying pan and fry the onions with the salt until softened – about 7–10 minutes.

Add the garlic, ginger and chillies and fry for a few more seconds. Add the spices and cook until you can smell them.

Add both types of tomato and stir through. Rinse out the can with a splash of water and add to the pan. Continue to cook for 15–20 minutes until the tomatoes have softened. Once cooked, the sauce can be blended to a smooth purée. Stir in the cream (if using – it can help with the heat if you find the sauce spicy and gives a velvety smooth finish) and coriander and season to taste. The sauce will keep in a sealed container in the fridge for up to 3 days.

SERVES 4

4 tablespoons ghee, butter or coconut oil
2 onions, finely chopped
1 teaspoon salt
3 garlic cloves, finely chopped
30g (1¼oz) fresh ginger, peeled and finely chopped
1–2 small green or red chillies, finely chopped, added according to taste
2 heaped teaspoons ground cumin
1 teaspoon ground turmeric
1 teaspoon chilli powder
2 teaspoons ground coriander
2 round tomatoes, finely diced
1 x 400g (14oz) can of plum tomatoes, chopped
3 tablespoons double cream (optional)
1 tablespoon chopped coriander

Per serving of curry base
14g carbs, 3g protein, 11g fat, 3.5g fibre, 179kcal

Masala Eggs

This is an easy and economical dish. We learnt to cook this in Calcutta and loved it so much that after a long night flight back from there, we cooked it for our breakfast when we got home.

Add the curry base to a large frying pan and bring to a gentle boil. Crack the eggs into the base and cook with the lid on until done – about 5 minutes.

Before serving, either dollop the yogurt on top, scatter over the herbs or shake over the dried mango powder, or use all three. Serve warm with lime wedges.

SERVES 4

1 quantity Masala Curry Base (see above)
8 eggs

To serve
4 tablespoons full-fat Greek yogurt
a handful of chopped coriander or parsley
1 teaspoon dried mango powder
4 lime wedges

Per serving 14g carbs, 17g protein, 19g fat, 3.7g fibre, 309kcal

Masala Vegetable Curry

We make this for our vegetarian friend Anne. It keeps well for a few days in the fridge and is easy to reheat and serve on its own, with cauliflower rice or halved boiled eggs. The chickpeas add protein but make the carbs higher so omit them if you are having eggs.

Preheat the oven to 200°C/fan 180°C/gas mark 6.

Mix together the oil, salt and a good pinch of black pepper in a large mixing bowl. Combine the vegetables and garlic with the oil using your hands and then spread them out on a baking tray.

Roast for 25 minutes or until tender and lightly browned at the edges.

Meanwhile, warm the masala curry base with the chickpeas (if using) in a large saucepan.

When the vegetables are cooked, remove from the oven and add to the curry sauce. Stir through and serve with coriander.

SERVES 4

4 tablespoons extra virgin olive oil
½ teaspoon salt
1 red pepper, cut into 2cm (¾in) dice
1 aubergine, cut into 2cm (¾in) dice
1 courgette, cut into 2cm (¾in) dice
1 onion, cut into 2cm (¾in) dice
3 garlic cloves, lightly crushed
1 quantity Masala Curry Base (see opposite) with the cream
1 x 400g (14oz) can of chickpeas, drained and rinsed (optional)
freshly ground black pepper
coriander leaves, to serve

Per serving 25g carbs, 8.4g protein, 22g fat, 9.3g fibre, 358kcal

Lentil-less Dal

This has all the comforting softness of a traditional dal but hardly any of the carbs. It is delicious served with curries or for breakfast or lunch with a couple of fried eggs. If I want to make it more presentable, I scatter over coriander or dollop on some Greek yogurt and mint leaves… delicious. Make sure you have all the ingredients ready before you begin as the recipe requires quick cooking at the start.

Heat the fat in a large frying pan over a high heat. Add the cumin seeds and dried chilli and fry for about 15 seconds. Add the garlic, stir through for a few seconds, then add the onion and stir again.

Reduce the temperature to medium, add the ginger and tomato and stir through. Let everything soften for a few minutes and then add the turmeric, lentils (if using), sprouts, paprika, green chilli and seasoning. Fry for a few minutes and then add the stock or water. Stir well and put the lid on.

Cook over a medium heat for 10–15 minutes, or until the riced sprouts have softened, stirring occasionally. It might need a little longer, and a little more stock, if you are using lentils.

Remove the chillies and blend with a stick blender or in a food-processor. Warm through in the pan and add a little more stock or water as necessary to get a thick, soupy consistency. Stir through the coriander leaves and serve straight away.

SERVES 8

3 tablespoons ghee, extra virgin olive oil or coconut oil

½ teaspoon cumin seeds

1 dried red chilli, stalk removed or pinch of chilli flakes

3 garlic cloves, grated

1 white onion, finely chopped

10g (¼oz) fresh ginger, peeled and grated

1 medium round tomato, finely chopped or coarsely grated

1 teaspoon ground turmeric

50g (2oz) dried red lentils, washed (optional)

600g (1lb 5oz) Brussels sprouts, cauliflower (leaves and head), Romanesco or broccoli, riced (see page 166)

1 teaspoon unsmoked paprika

1 green chilli, split

salt and freshly ground black pepper

600ml (20fl oz) hot vegetable stock or water, plus up to 100ml (3½fl oz) to finish

small bunch coriander, leaves roughly chopped, stems finely chopped, to serve

Per 122g serving without lentils
5.6g carbs, 3.2g protein, 6.2g fat, 3.7g fibre, 99kcal

Per 125g serving with lentils
6.5g carbs, 3.6g protein, 6.2g fat, 4g fibre, 105kcal

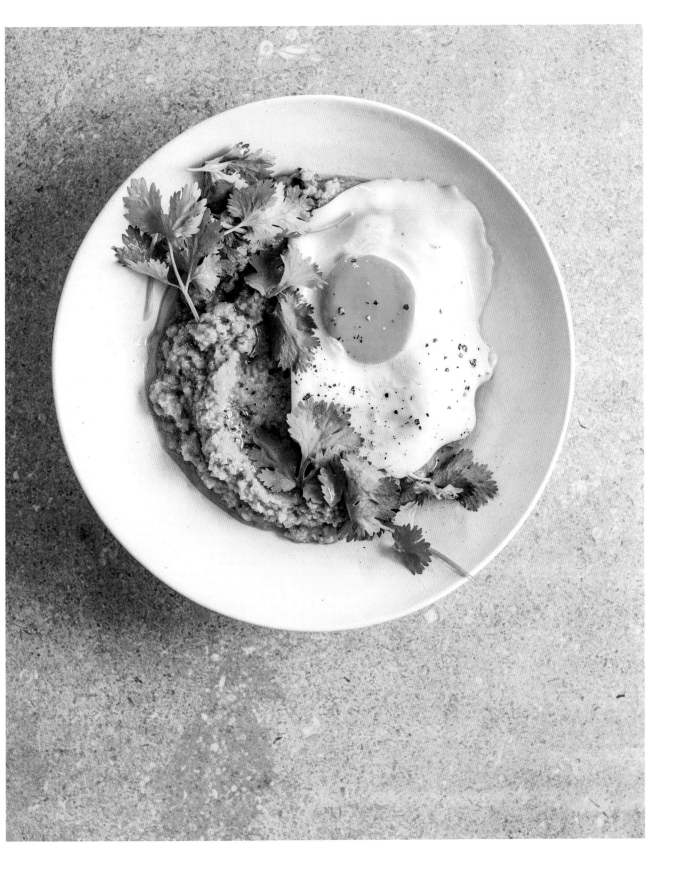

Cauliflower Rice

If only our local curry house sold cauliflower rice I would be the first to order it – I'm sure it is only a matter of time. Until then I can make the rice in the time it takes for a curry to arrive so I am not tempted to order white rice and naan. You can microwave or roast cauliflower rice, but we prefer to stir-fry it so that you can add other flavours to it at the same time. It keeps well once cooked in the fridge for up to 3 days (or in the freezer for up to 3 months), so leftovers are quick to reheat. Broccoli or Romanesco rice can be made in the same way or use both vegetables mixed together.

Basic Cauliflower Rice

This is a simple way to prepare cauliflower rice and an excellent substitute for simple white rice. To add a little zing and colour, add the zest of a lemon or a handful of chopped flat-leaf parsley or coriander. Use this recipe on its own or combine it with the recipes below or opposite to take it in a different direction.

Cut the head of the cauliflower into florets and roughly chop the stalk and leaves. Put a third of the cauliflower into a food-processor and pulse until finely chopped (it will resemble large grains of rice), making sure you don't end up with a purée. Tip into a bowl and repeat with the remaining two thirds. Alternatively, coarsely grate the florets and stalk and finely chop the leaves.

Heat the fat in a wok or large frying pan. Fry the onion over a medium heat for 7 minutes or until soft. Add the cauliflower rice, hot water and seasoning and stir through. Cover and cook over a low heat, stirring occasionally, for about 7 minutes, or until just soft.

SERVES 6

800g–1kg (1¾lb–2¼lb) cauliflower (head stalk and leaves)
4 tablespoons extra virgin olive oil, ghee, coconut oil, chicken fat or beef dripping
1 onion, finely chopped, or 5 spring onions, finely chopped
6 tablespoons hot water
1 teaspoon salt
freshly ground black pepper

Per serving *12g carbs, 4g protein, 8.9g fat, 3.2g fibre, 146kcal*

Indian Cauliflower Pilao

We love this with our curries and use the traditional spices used to make pilao rice.

Heat the ghee in a frying pan. Add the spices and cook until they splutter. Follow the recipe for Basic Cauliflower Rice (see above) adding the fried spices to the onion once it is cooked.

SERVES 6

4 tablespoons ghee
1 teaspoon cumin seeds
5 cloves
5 cardamom pods, lightly crushed
2 bay leaves
1 small cinnamon stick

Values as above per serving

Southeast Asian Cauliflower Rice

This is great served with Thai Green Curry (page 120).

Dry-fry the coconut (if using) in a wok or frying pan until golden brown. Transfer to a plate and set aside.

Follow the recipe for Basic Cauliflower Rice (see opposite) using coconut oil and add the garlic, ginger and chilli to the onion. Mix in the coriander (if using). Serve scattered with the coriander (if using).

SERVES 6

3 tablespoons desiccated coconut (optional)
3 garlic cloves, coarsely chopped
thumb-sized piece of fresh ginger, peeled and finely chopped
1 red hot chilli (according to taste), finely chopped
10g (¼oz) coriander, leaves roughly chopped and stems finely chopped (optional)

Per serving 13g carbs, 4.3g protein, 11g fat, 4.1g fibre, 172kcal

Middle Eastern Cauliflower Rice

This brightly-coloured fragrant dish is perfect with Kuwaiti Spiced Lamb Shoulder (page 118) as well as any roast meats or dishes that have a Middle Eastern, Greek or Spanish vibe.

Preheat the oven to 200°C/fan 180°C/gas mark 6.

Put the saffron threads into a small bowl with the hot water and set aside.

Spread the almonds out on a baking tray and toast them in the oven for 6 minutes or until lightly browned. Leave to cool.

Put the aubergine, onion and garlic into a bowl with 3 tablespoons of the oil and some seasoning. Toss through and lay onto a baking tray, making sure the vegetables are in a single layer and not in piles otherwise they will steam and not crisp up. Roast for 25 minutes.

Pour the remaining oil into a large, non-stick frying pan or wok and add the chilli flakes, cauliflower rice, saffron threads and water, spices and almonds, and season. Keep stirring the cauliflower as it cooks. Add the roast aubergine and onion. Squeeze out the garlic cloves, roughly chop and add them to the pan. Season to taste.

Stir in the herbs and serve straight away.

SERVES 6

½ teaspoon saffron threads
2 tablespoons hot water
3 tablespoons flaked almonds
1 aubergine, cut into 2cm (¾in) cubes
1 red onion, cut into 2cm (¾in) cubes
2 garlic cloves, peeled
6 tablespoons extra virgin olive oil
¼ teaspoon chilli flakes
800g–1kg (1¾lb–2¼lb) cauliflower, riced (see opposite)
½ teaspoon ground cumin
½ teaspoon ground turmeric
a large handful of dill, roughly chopped
a large handful of coriander or parsley, leaves roughly chopped and stems finely chopped
salt and freshly ground black pepper

Per serving 8.3g carbs, 6.2g protein, 19g fat, 5.1g fibre, 259kcal

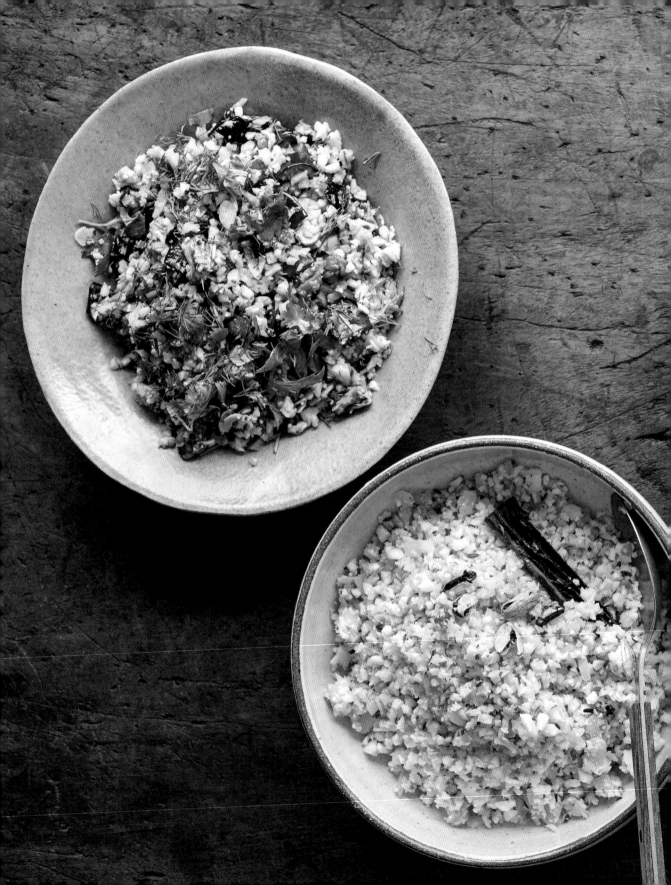

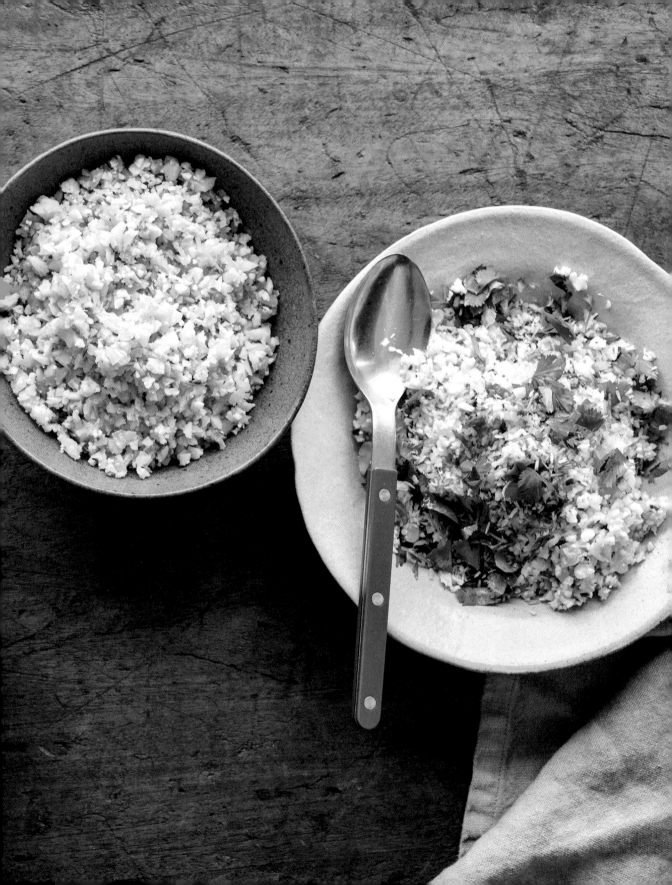

Mash!

Years ago, I would never have imagined another kind of mash other than potato, or perhaps swede at Christmas. Now we have a rainbow of mash to choose from made with low-carb vegetables, such as cauliflower, celeriac, pumpkin, squash, swede, carrot, Brussels sprouts and broccoli. I love their individual flavours and what they bring to the party. Celeriac is good with meat as well as fish; while cauliflower and swede are better with meat, sausages and eggs.

Some can be made with a potato masher, while others need a little more persuasion with the aid of a food-processor or stick blender to transform their fibrous nature into the creamy result we all love. Any leftovers keep well in the fridge and make a good base for eggs the next day.

Cauliflower Mash

By using the leaves and stalks of a cauliflower you get a lot more mash for your money and the taste is the same. Since the stalks will take longer to cook, cut them into smaller pieces than the florets and leaves.

Steam or boil the cauliflower until it is just tender. Drain well.

Blend with the butter, milk, salt and a good pinch of pepper in a food-processor or with a stick blender until smooth. Season to taste. Spoon into a warm bowl and dot with extra butter to serve.

SERVES 4

800g (1¾lb) cauliflower florets, stalks and leaves, roughly chopped
50g (2oz) salted butter or extra virgin olive oil, plus extra to serve
100ml (3½fl oz) nut or cow's milk
½ teaspoon salt
freshly ground black pepper

Per serving 7.1g carbs, 4.2g protein, 12g fat, 3.8g fibre, 164kcal

Flavourings

Add one of the following to the mash for a change:
- 100g (3½oz) feta, coarsely grated
- 50g (2oz) Parmesan, finely grated, plus more to top
- 1 heaped teaspoon mustard powder
- 1–2 tablespoons horseradish sauce (according to taste)
- 4 tablespoons pesto (page 122)
- 4 tablespoons double or soured cream, or crème fraîche

BROCCOLI Follow the instructions above, substituting the cauliflower for broccoli.
Per serving 6.1g carbs, 6.8g protein, 12g fat, 5.6g fibre, 166kcal

BRUSSELS SPROUTS Follow the instructions above allowing a few minutes longer for the sprouts to cook.
Per serving 7.2g carbs, 6.1g protein, 13g fat, 5.2g fibre, 182kcal

CELERIAC (see Fish Pie page 139)
Per serving 4.7g carbs, 2.8g protein, 11g fat, 7.4g fibre, 146kcal

SWEDE
Per serving 4.7g carbs, 0.9g protein, 11g fat, 1.4g fibre, 122kcal

Celeriac Dauphinoise

Jenny Phillips once disclosed to me that she would choose any dish from a restaurant menu as long as it had potato dauphinoise with it! Never mind what kind of meat it was; it was all about the creamy, garlicky side. Jen Unwin showed us this version swapping the potatoes for low-carb celeriac, so now we can all enjoy this indulgent classic with roast meats, sausages or fish, or on its own.

Preheat the oven to 200°C/fan 180°C/gas mark 6.

Mix together the cream, garlic, nutmeg, butter and seasoning in a bowl. Put a layer of celeriac slices into an ovenproof dish — we use a round one with a 25cm (10in) diameter and approx. 6cm (2½in) deep, but any similar size will work. Pour over a layer of the cream. Repeat this until both the celeriac and cream are used up, finishing with the cream.

Cover with foil to avoid it drying out and bake for 30 minutes. Remove the foil and let it brown for a further 15 minutes, or until the celeriac is tender when pierced with a knife. Leave to stand for 10 minutes before serving.

SERVES 8

300ml (10fl oz) double cream
3 fat garlic cloves, finely chopped
½ teaspoon freshly grated nutmeg
100g (3½oz) butter, melted
800g–1kg (1¾lb–2¼lb) celeriac,
   peeled, quartered and finely sliced
salt and freshly ground black pepper

Per serving 3.7g carbs,
2.3g protein, 31g fat, 4.7g fibre,
311kcal

Chips

Steak and chips, fish and chips, burger and chips — we are a nation of chip lovers. Since potatoes are out on a low-carb diet we have come up with some even-better-than-the-spud alternatives packed with colour and flavour. They are triple-fried to get the best results and increase the resistant starch. We have used roots but even the stems of cauliflower leaves make excellent chips. To give you some carb comparisons per 100g (3½oz) fried chips: sweet potatoes contain 20g carbs, white potatoes 18g, parsnips 12g, carrots 7g, swede 5g and the lowest of all celeriac has just 2.3g.

Heat the fat to 180°C (350°F) in either a deep-fat fryer or a high-sided saucepan and fry the chips for 2 minutes or until very lightly browned. Remove with a slotted spoon and set aside on kitchen paper until cool to the touch.

Fry as above for a further 1–2 minutes until slightly darker and set aside as before.

Just before you are ready to serve, fry for the last time for a further 1–2 minutes or until golden brown all over and the vegetables are cooked through. Serve straight away scattered with salt to taste.

SERVES 4

500g root vegetables, such as swede,
   celeriac, parsnips, carrots and
   turnips, cut into chips (100g of
   each)
lard, beef dripping, duck fat, goose fat
   or coconut oil for shallow or deep
   frying
salt

Per serving 7.8g carbs,
1.3g protein, 1.9g fat, 4.3g fibre,
62kcal

Green Stir-fry

This is our go-to quick and crunchy stir-fry to have in place of rice. The low-carb vegetables used will vary throughout the year, but keep to those that grow above the ground and always include some herbs. Nuts are good to add for texture and to bump up the satiety, and any stir-fry can be made into a main meal with eggs, meat, fish or tofu thrown in.

Prepare the cabbage by cutting it into slices about 3mm thick with a large, sharp knife. Lay a few of these onto a board on top of one another and slice down thinly to make long, thin strips.

Heat the ghee or oil in a large wok or non-stick frying pan. When hot, add the vegetables and stir constantly, keeping the pan over a high heat for 4–5 minutes until the vegetables become tender but still have some bite.

Stir in the butter and dill (if using) and serve straight away.

SERVES 4

100g (3½oz) white or green cabbage, outer leaves discarded
2 tablespoons ghee, extra virgin olive oil or reserved chicken or beef fat
2 spring onions, finely sliced
150g (5oz) fennel, finely sliced
200g (7oz) sugar snap peas, finely sliced
1 garlic clove, finely chopped
10g (¼oz) butter
a small handful of dill, roughly chopped (optional)
salt and freshly ground black pepper

Per serving 4.5g carbs, 2.9g protein, 16g fat, 3.3g fibre, 180kcal

Chinese Green Stir-fry

Enjoy this on its own or with it goes well with Chinese duck dishes. It's easy and much healthier than resorting to using a pre-made sauce packed with sugar.

Heat the fat in a large wok or non-stick frying pan. When hot, add the chilli, garlic and ginger. Fry for 2 minutes, then add the spring onions. Fry for a further 2 minutes and then add the green vegetables. Stir constantly, keeping the pan over a high heat for 4–5 minutes until the vegetables become tender but still have some bite.

Stir in the soy sauce, rice wine and sesame oil. Stir in the eggs (if using) and serve scattered with sesame seeds.

SERVES 2

2 tablespoons untoasted sesame oil, ghee or reserved chicken or beef fat
1 hot green or red chilli, finely chopped
2 fat garlic cloves, finely grated
15g (½oz) fresh ginger, peeled and finely grated
5 spring onions, finely sliced
500g (18oz) mixed green vegetables, such as mangetout, green pepper, green beans, pak choi, broccoli, finely sliced
2 tablespoons soy sauce
2 tablespoons rice wine or dry sherry
1 teaspoon toasted sesame oil
2 eggs, beaten (optional)
1 tablespoon toasted sesame seeds

Per serving 18g carbs, 18g protein, 24g fat, 8.2g fibre, 388kcal

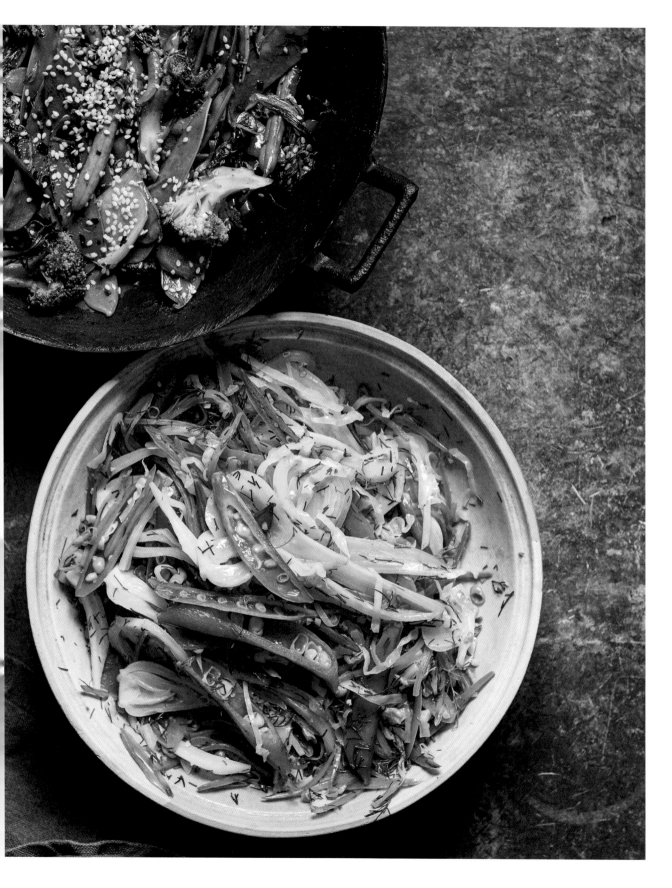

Spicy Paneer with Curry Leaves & Gravy

This wonderful curry was shown to us by the passionate chefs from Mrs Magpie cafe in Calcutta, run by our friend Sohini Basu. The chefs called the sauce gravy and make the same curry with prawns or chicken breast. Do seek out fresh curry leaves (dried leaves have no flavour) – they can be found in Asian shops or online and will freeze well.

Heat the fat in a large frying pan. Fry the paneer cubes over a medium heat until golden brown on most sides. Remove from the pan and set aside.

To prepare the marinade, heat the fat in the same pan and fry the curry leaves, chillies, almonds and spices for 2 minutes until they splutter. Remove from the heat and tip the contents of the pan into a blender. Add the remaining marinade ingredients with 2 tablespoons of cold water and blitz quickly until crushed, but still retaining some texture.

Remove 2 heaped tablespoons of the marinade and set aside for the gravy. Spoon the remaining paste into a large bowl and add the paneer. Toss to mix. Leave to infuse for 30 minutes (or up to overnight) in the fridge.

Meanwhile, make the gravy. Heat the fat in a frying pan and fry the marinade paste for a couple of minutes. Add the tomatoes and tamarind paste or lemon juice and cook for 2 minutes before adding the stock or water. Bring to the boil, then reduce the heat and simmer until the gravy is reduced by a third. Season with salt to taste.

Add the marinated paneer to the gravy and stir to combine. Serve straight away on its own or with Indian Cauliflower Pilao (page 166) scattered with coriander.

SERVES 4

2 tablespoons butter or ghee
600g (1lb 5oz) paneer, cut into approx. 2cm (¾in) cubes
1 teaspoon coriander, leaves roughly chopped and stems finely chopped, to serve

For the marinade

3 tablespoons ghee, butter or extra virgin olive oil
a large handful of fresh curry leaves, pulled off the stalk
4 dried red chillies
50g (2oz) almonds, roughly chopped
2 teaspoons mustard seeds
½ teaspoon fenugreek seeds
2 teaspoons coriander seeds
½ teaspoon ground cumin
1 teaspoon salt
5 fat garlic cloves, peeled

For the gravy

20g (¾oz) ghee, butter or extra virgin olive oil
100g (3½oz) tomatoes (approx. 3 round tomatoes), finely diced
2 teaspoons tamarind paste/ concentrate or lemon juice
300ml (10fl oz) hot vegetable stock or water
salt

Per serving 5.2g carbs, 40g protein, 50g fat, 1.5g fibre, 650kcal

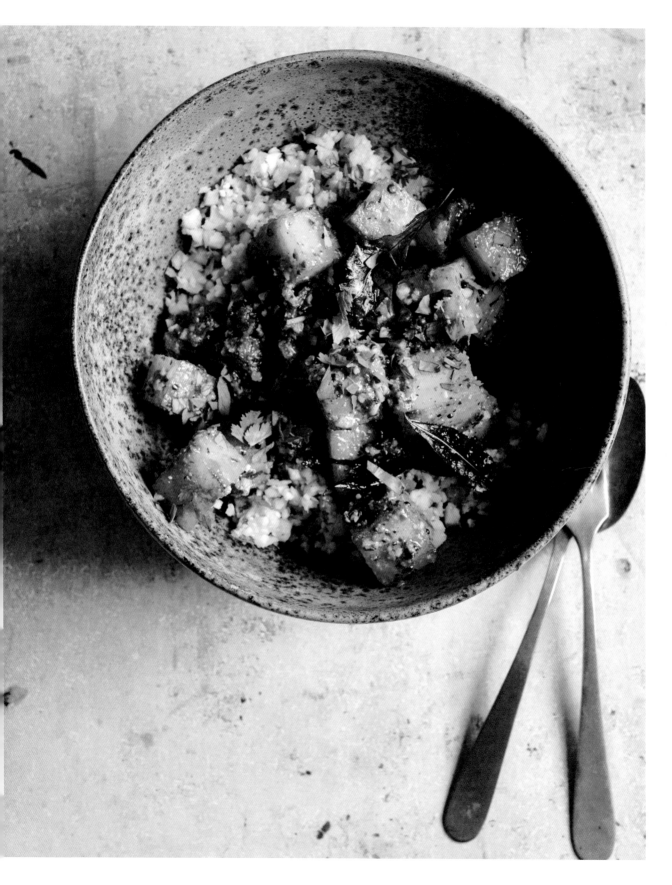

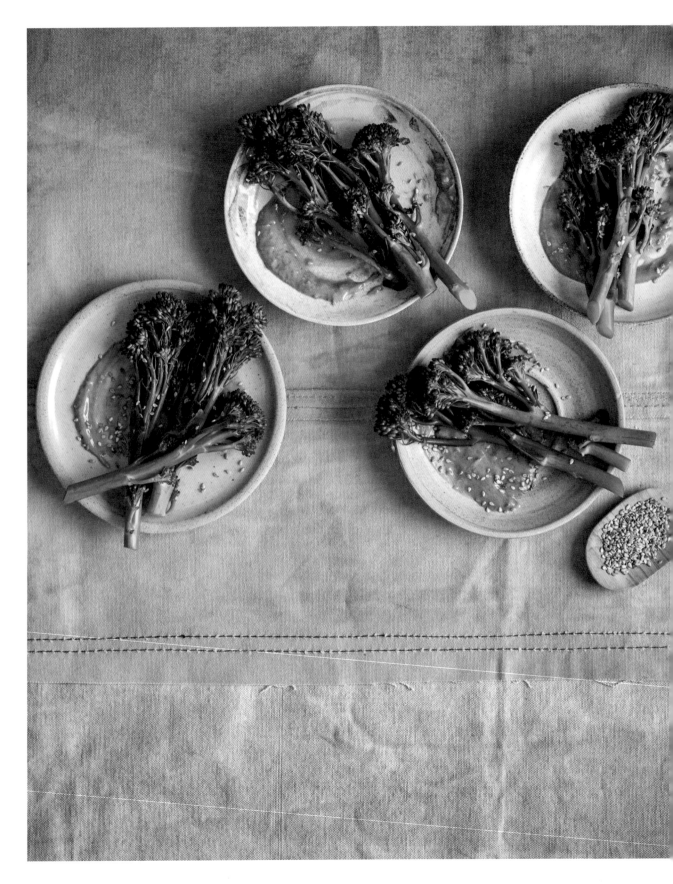

Broccoli Spears with Ginger, Soy & Peanut Dressing

Warm stems of broccoli are the perfect vegetable for this spicy, nutty dip as it clings to the bumpy, uneven heads. Cauliflower florets also work well. We rustle this up as a starter if we have friends round, or for a quick bite for hungry boys. It could also be a light meal on its own with boiled eggs.

Whisk the dressing ingredients together in a small bowl and adjust the balance of flavours accordingly. The dressing will keep well in a sealed jar in the fridge for up to 3 days.

If any broccoli stems are thick, split them in half by making a cut halfway up from the base to allow the heat to penetrate. Boil or steam the broccoli until soft – around 5 minutes.

Put some dressing in small bowls or on each plate. Arrange the broccoli around it and scatter over the sesame seeds. Serve while the broccoli is still warm.

SERVES 4

200g (7oz) broccoli or Tenderstem broccoli spears
2 teaspoons toasted sesame seeds, to serve

For the dressing

2 tablespoons sesame oil (not toasted) or extra virgin olive oil
2 tablespoons tamari or soy sauce
3 tablespoons lime juice or rice wine vinegar
10g (¼oz) fresh ginger, peeled and finely grated
1 garlic clove, finely grated
1 small green chilli (according to taste), finely sliced
3 tablespoons smooth or crunchy peanut butter
1 teaspoon toasted sesame oil
2 teaspoons sesame seeds, toasted
1 teaspoon clear honey

Per serving 5.8g carbs, 6.9g protein, 16g fat, 2.8g fibre, 200kcal

Horta with Lemon & Oil

I discovered "horta" – a mixture of seasonal soft green leaves – on a trip to Greece. Most cultures have a variation on this dish: the Italians add oil, chilli and garlic; the French add cream; the Indians add ghee. Horta makes a quick meal with eggs, fish or meat, or try my favourite addition of roasted red peppers and fried cubes of halloumi cheese.

Pull the green leaves away from any tough stalks and wash them under cold water. Roughly shred the leaves and put them in a steamer or in a pan of salted boiling water for a few minutes until cooked and tender. Drain the leaves of any excess water, but don't squeeze them dry.

Toss the leaves with the oil and a generous pinch of salt and black pepper, squeeze over the lemon juice and serve.

SERVES 4

1kg (2¼lb) mixed soft green leaves, such as spinach, rocket, chard, watercress
3 tablespoons extra virgin olive oil
juice of 1 lemon
salt and freshly ground black pepper

Per serving 4.2g carbs, 7.1g protein, 11g fat, 9.1g fibre, 165kcal

Variations

WINTER GREENS WITH LEMON & OIL
Use firm green leaves, such as kale, cavolo nero, curly kale or green cabbage, and follow the recipe above.

SAUTÉED GREENS WITH CHILLI & GARLIC
Follow the recipe above until the leaves are drained. Fry a little finely sliced chilli and 2 crushed garlic cloves in the oil for a couple of minutes before adding the leaves. Serve warm. Omit the lemon juice.

Cheat's Creamy Spinach

This is the French way to eat spinach and it is utterly delicious in under 10 minutes! If you don't have a microwave, defrost and drain the spinach before adding to a pan with remaining ingredients and heat through.

Put the spinach in a small plastic or glass bowl. Cook it in the microwave on full power for 7 minutes or until defrosted. Tip it into a sieve and use the base of the bowl to push down on the spinach squeezing the water through the sieve. Rinse the bottom of the bowl and tip the spinach back inside.
Add the butter, cream, nutmeg and seasoning to the bowl, stir through and put back into the microwave on full power for a further 2 minutes, or until hot. Season to taste.

SERVES 4

1kg (2¼lb) frozen chopped spinach
25g (1oz) salted butter
100ml (3½fl oz) double cream
¼ teaspoon freshly grated nutmeg
salt and freshly ground black pepper

Per 180g serving 1.3g carbs, 5.1g protein, 19g fat, 4.8g fibre, 207kcal

Saag

Pratima Basu – the owner of a chain of Hyderabadi restaurants in Calcutta called Khawab – taught me her way of cooking this spicy spinach dish. Pratima has type 2 diabetes and this is one of her favourite dishes to make at home. I love to cook a batch of it as it keeps well in the fridge. Instead of serving it with the traditional rice, try it with Cauliflower Rice (page 166).

Drain the spinach of most of the excess water, but don't squeeze it dry.

Heat the fat in a large, non-stick frying pan. Gently fry the onion with the salt until soft. Add the garlic, chillies and ginger and fry for 1 minute. Add the spices and let them sizzle, frying for a further 2 minutes.

Chop the spinach with scissors if it isn't already chopped. Add to the pan with the tomatoes and coriander (if using); if it looks dry, add a splash of water to the pan. Cover and cook for 15 minutes. Add the cream and stir through. Season to taste.

SERVES 6

600g (1lb 5oz) spinach (from approx. 2kg/4½lb frozen spinach), defrosted (drained weight)
4 tablespoons ghee, butter or extra virgin olive oil
1 onion, finely chopped
1 teaspoon salt
4 fat garlic cloves, roughly chopped
1–2 fine green chillies (according to taste), finely chopped, or ½ teaspoon chilli flakes
25g (1oz) fresh ginger, peeled and finely chopped
1 teaspoon ground cumin
1 teaspoon fenugreek seeds, crushed
¼ teaspoon ground turmeric
3 round tomatoes, finely diced
25g (1oz) coriander leaves (optional)
5 tablespoons double cream

Per serving *6.4g carbs, 4.8g protein, 17g fat, 4.9g fibre, 206kcal*

Buttered Medley of Green Vegetables

This stunning collection of green vegetables shines with butter and health. Serve as it is or add a little lemon zest for zing, a little chilli for a kick and a handful of herbs for flavour.
Bring a large saucepan of salted water to the boil. Put the vegetables with the longest cooking time into the water first, such as green beans and asparagus. After a couple of minutes, add the softer vegetables, such as mangetout and peas. Cook until the vegetables are tender, and then drain.

Melt the butter in a large pan or wok over a medium heat, add the cooked vegetables and use tongs to combine. Season to taste and serve straight away.

SERVES 6

1kg (2¼lb) mixed green vegetables, such as green beans, asparagus, mangetout, sugar snap peas
125g (4½oz) salted butter, at room temperature
salt and freshly ground black pepper

Per serving *6g carbs, 5.1g protein, 18g fat, 3.7g fibre, 211kcal*

Steamed Vegetable Parcels

Steamed vegetables can be boring but with just another few minutes of tender loving care everyday vegetables can be transformed into a glorious array of colour, texture, flavour and excitement. Some examples of flavourings and timings are below. Let children and fussy eaters prepare their own parcels (and name them) and generally just have fun with flavour. Cooking the vegetables "al cartoccio" (in paper parcels) means that the juices are kept in the parcel, so go easy with the seasoning.

- *Courgettes, thinly sliced, with extra virgin olive oil: 7–10 minutes*
- *Leeks, cut into 1cm (½in) discs, cherry tomatoes and a knob of butter: 8 minutes*
- *Shredded savoy cabbage with ghee, salt, cumin seeds and garam masala: 8–10 minutes*
- *Cauliflower florets with black pepper, black onion seeds, salt, garlic and butter: 15 minutes*
- *Thinly sliced fennel with a splash of white wine, butter and a few fennel seeds: 12 minutes*
- *Carrot batons and chopped leeks with salted butter and dill or tarragon: 20–35 minutes*

Preheat the oven to 180°C/fan 160°C/gas mark 4.

To make a cartoccio, or parcel, cut a piece of baking parchment at least 10cm (4in) larger all around than the food you are about to cook. Lay the vegetables in the centre of the paper. Bring the long ends up to meet each other above the food, then fold together making a finger-width closure. Fold several more times until the fold is about 4cm (1½in) above the food. Now twist the short ends like a sweet. Place the parcel on a baking tray to cook according to the timings above. Press the top of the parcels to feel if the vegetables are cooked to your liking.

Variation

DR UNWIN'S STEAMED VEGETABLES
Another way to steam the vegetables, shown to me by Dr David Unwin, is to fill a small microwaveproof container with bite-sized pieces of vegetables, such as peppers, courgettes and beans. If he has leftover meat, he adds that, too. Season and add 1 tablespoon of extra virgin olive oil. The container can then be microwaved at work for a filling and healthy lunch.

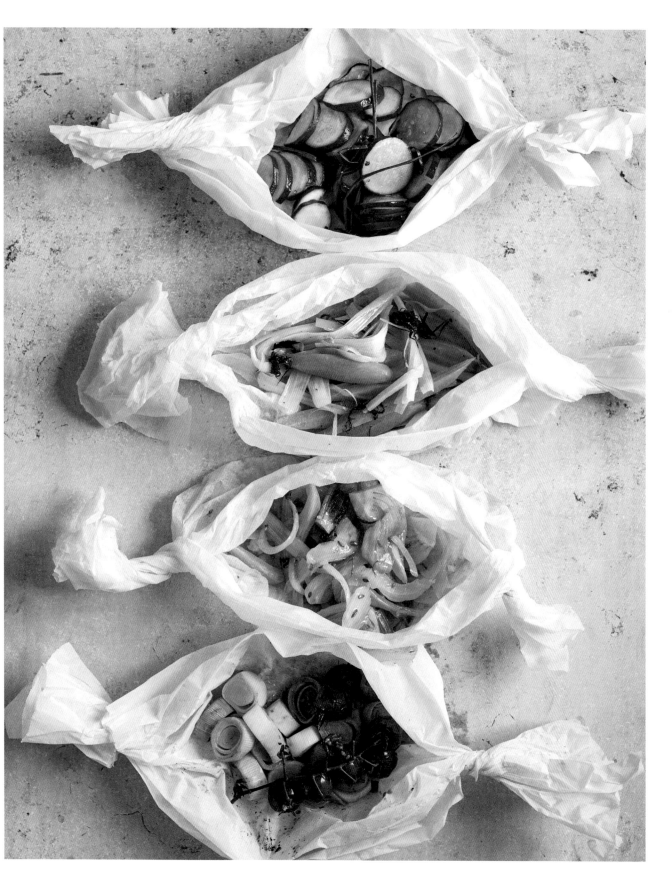

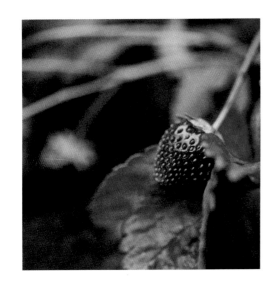

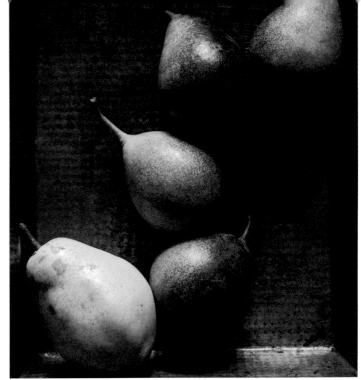

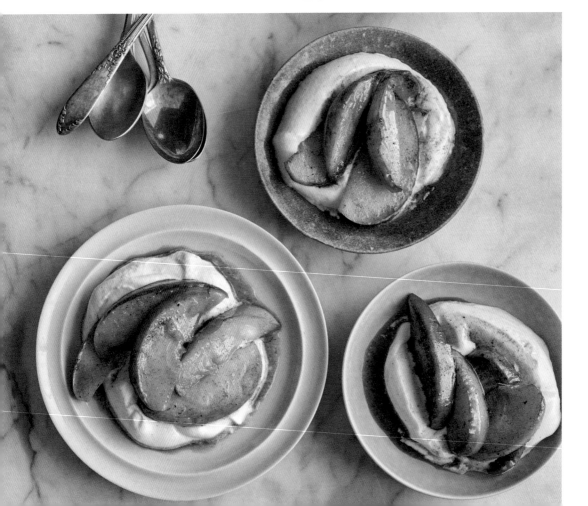

Petite PUDDINGS

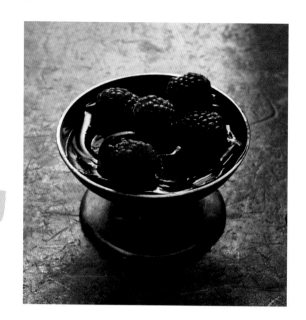

As a sugar addict, Giancarlo hasn't lost his sweet tooth completely, but his taste has changed. Commercial ice cream and cakes are just too sweet for his altered taste buds. After a long day at the restaurants, his way to relax is with a black coffee in front of the football and a small square of either of the low-carb cakes on pages 184 and 186.

There will always be occasions when you want to share a treat with family and friends. In this chapter, we have devised some healthier recipes that are every bit as indulgent and flavourful as standard puddings but with none of the harmful sugar. We don't add artificial sweeteners as we don't like the idea of ultra-processed food and most of the time they have an unpleasant flavour. Instead we use vanilla, apples, pears and minimal dates when a little sweetness is desired.

The Magic Muffins (page 77) can be adapted to form a scone-like base for cream, jam and berries, or you can make mini versions to have with coffee. The Greek Yogurt with Blueberries, Cinnamon Granola & Raspberry Jam (page 63) is also great as a dessert.

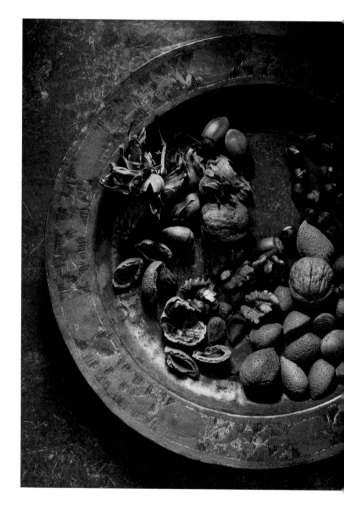

Hot Chocolate Pots

This recipe is a chocoholic's idea of heaven, as our son Giorgio will vouch. If you pour out a couple of small cups for the children, you can then add a shot of booze to the remaining for the grown-ups! And if you don't mind a slightly bitter taste, leave out the date to reduce the carbs even further.

Melt the date in 3 tablespoons of the milk in a cup in the microwave on full power for 1 minute, or in a small pan over a medium heat. It will become soft and can be mashed with a fork. Put this mixture into a sieve and push it through with a spoon into a medium saucepan. Discard the skin of the date.

Add the remaining milk to the pan with the cream and egg yolks and whisk to combine. Put over a medium heat and bring almost to boiling point, stirring constantly. It needs to reach 85°C (185°F) to sterilize and thicken the custard. If you don't have a thermometer, check that the custard coats the back of a wooden spoon and, if you run your finger through it, the line remains visible.

Remove from the heat, add the chocolate and whisk to melt. It will look lumpy to begin with but will soon become velvety smooth. Add the rum (if using).

Serve in warm espresso cups while still hot. You can drink it, dip strawberries into it or serve it with a spoonful of whipped cream. If left to cool in the fridge, the chocolate will set and can be eaten the following day.

SERVES 4

½ Medjool date, stoned and halved
120ml (4fl oz) almond milk
100ml (3½fl oz) double cream
2 egg yolks
150g (5oz) good-quality dark chocolate (minimum 85 per cent cocoa solids), coarsely grated or cut into very small pieces
3 tablespoons rum or brandy (optional)

Per serving 12g carbs, 5.5g protein, 37g fat, 4.8g fibre, 434kcal

Orange & Almond Cake

We love this flavourful cake topped with mascarpone or Greek yogurt. It is rich with the almonds so enjoy it in small portions. Serve with crème fraîche or mascarpone and Raspberry Chia Jam (page 63) or fresh berries.

Put the oranges into a medium saucepan and cover with hot water. Bring to the boil, then reduce the heat to a simmer. Cook for 2 hours. Remove the oranges from the water and leave to cool. Discard the water.

Preheat the oven to 190°C/fan 170°C/gas mark 5. Line a 23 x 26cm (9 x10½in) cake tin with baking parchment or grease it well.

Slice the oranges into quarters and remove any pips. Drop the oranges and dates into a food-processor and whizz until you have a purée. Add the remaining ingredients and whizz again until smooth. Spoon the mixture into the cake tin and smooth the surface. Bake for 40 minutes, or until firm and lightly browned. Leave to cool before removing from the tin and serving.

MAKES 1 CAKE/SERVES 10

2 oranges, washed in warm water
100g (3½oz) salted butter, at room temperature, plus extra to grease
3 Medjool dates, stoned
1 heaped teaspoon baking powder
300g (10½oz) ground almonds
4 eggs

Per serving 9.7g carbs, 6.8g protein, 17g fat, 4.8g fibre, 229kcal

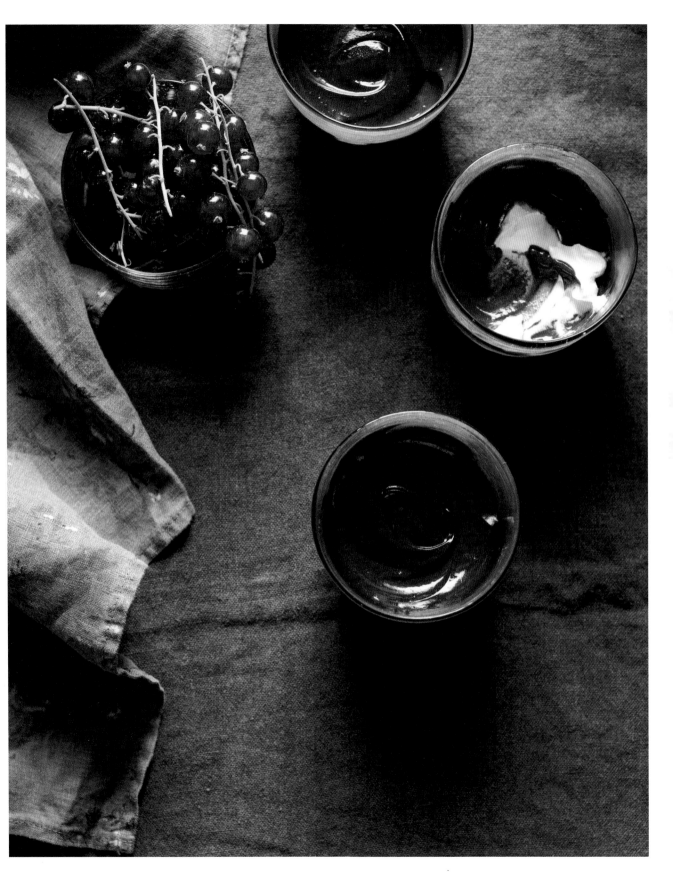

Peanut Butter & Jelly Cake

This decadent, irresistible cake was dreamt up by Jen Unwin as something to serve at celebrations while keeping low-carb. Feel free to swap the raspberries for strawberries when they are in season.

Preheat the oven to 200°C/fan 180°C/gas mark 6. Grease two 20cm (8in) round cake tins and cut a circle of baking parchment to fit the bottom of each one.

Mix the ground almonds and baking powder together in a large mixing bowl. In a separate bowl, mash the banana, butter and peanut butter together with a fork and then combine with the eggs and vanilla extract. Pour this mixture into the almonds and stir together with a large metal spoon.

Evenly divide the mixture between the two tins, level the tops and bake for 25 minutes, or until firm and a skewer inserted in the centre comes out clean. Remove the tins from the oven and leave to cool for 5 minutes before turning the cakes out onto a wire rack to cool completely.

Meanwhile, make the filling and topping. Whip the double cream and vanilla extract together with an electric or hand whisk until soft peaks form.

When the cakes are cool, spread the top of each one with 3 tablespoons of peanut butter. Spread half of the jam onto the surface of one followed by half the cream. Turn the other cake over, sandwiching both layers of peanut butter and the jam and cream inside. Transfer to a serving plate, top with the remaining cream and the raspberries and enjoy with the remaining jam in a bowl on the side. The cake will keep, covered, in the fridge for up to 3 days.

MAKES 1 CAKE/SERVES 10

150g (5oz) butter, plus extra to grease
300g (10½oz) ground almonds
2 teaspoons baking powder
1 medium banana, peeled
100g (3½oz) crunchy peanut butter
4 large eggs
2 teaspoons vanilla extract

For the cream filling and topping
300ml (10fl oz) double cream
1 teaspoon vanilla extract
6 tablespoons crunchy peanut butter
1 quantity Raspberry Chia Jam (page 63)

To serve
a handful of raspberries

Per serving 9.6g carbs, 16g protein, 55g fat, 9.3g fibre, 618kcal

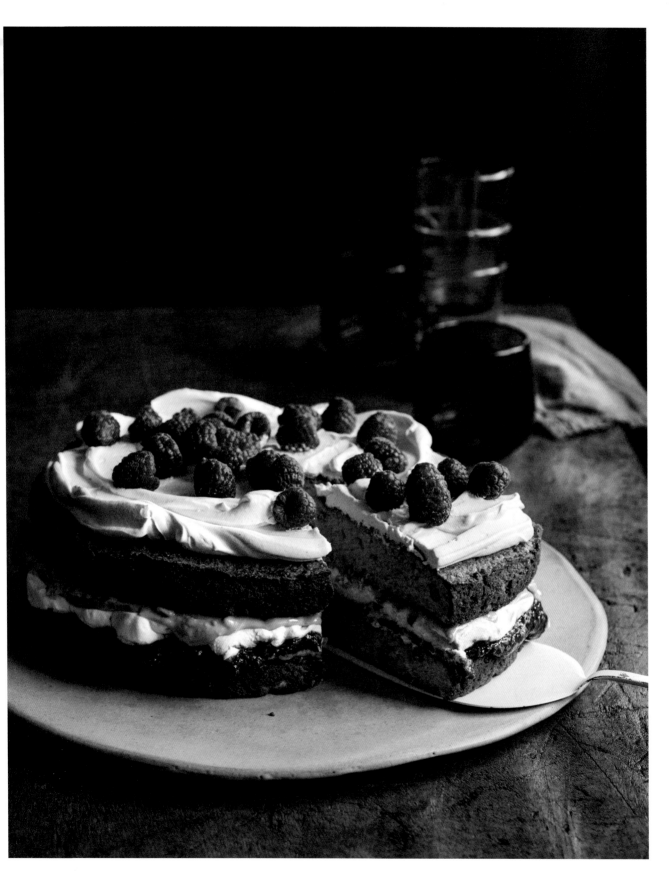

Cinnamon & Brandy Buttered Apples & Whipped Vanilla Cream

These apples are the perfect comfort dish served with whipped cream or Greek yogurt.

Slice the apples into quarters, leaving the skin on, and remove the core from each part. Cut each quarter into four slices.

For the whipped vanilla cream, whip the cream and vanilla extract together until thick in a large bowl by hand or with an electric whisk.

Melt the butter in a non-stick frying pan and, when bubbling, add the apple. Let the apples brown on one side and then flip over with a spatula. Scatter over the cinnamon and pour over the brandy (if using) and water and continue to cook for 7–10 minutes, or until soft. Serve straight away or keep warm until needed, and serve with dollops of whipped vanilla cream on the side.

SERVES 4

3 medium dessert apples
60g (2¼oz) salted butter
1 teaspoon ground cinnamon
100ml (3½fl oz) brandy (optional)
3 tablespoons hot water

For the whipped vanilla cream
300ml (10fl oz) whipping cream
3 teaspoons vanilla extract

Per serving of buttered apples
14g carbs, 0.7g protein, 13g fat, 1.3g fibre, 237kcal
Per serving of whipped cream
2g carbs, 1.5g protein, 30g fat, 0g fibre, 287kcal

Quick Raspberry & Mascarpone Ice Cream

Giancarlo always loved gelato when we were in Italy. Now we find ice cream too sweet so prefer to make our own without sugar, just using the natural sweetness from the fruit.

We love raspberries in our family, so I frequently buy them when they are on offer and freeze them. This is a super quick way to make ice cream shown to me by Jen Unwin. If the fruit is very tart, then add a soft stoned Medjool date to the mix.

Whizz all the ingredients together in a food-processor and serve straight away in chilled glasses.

SERVES 4

225–250g (8–9oz) frozen raspberries
250g (9oz) mascarpone
2 teaspoons vanilla extract

Per serving *5.5g carbs, 3.6g protein, 28g fat, 3.6g fibre, 301kcal*

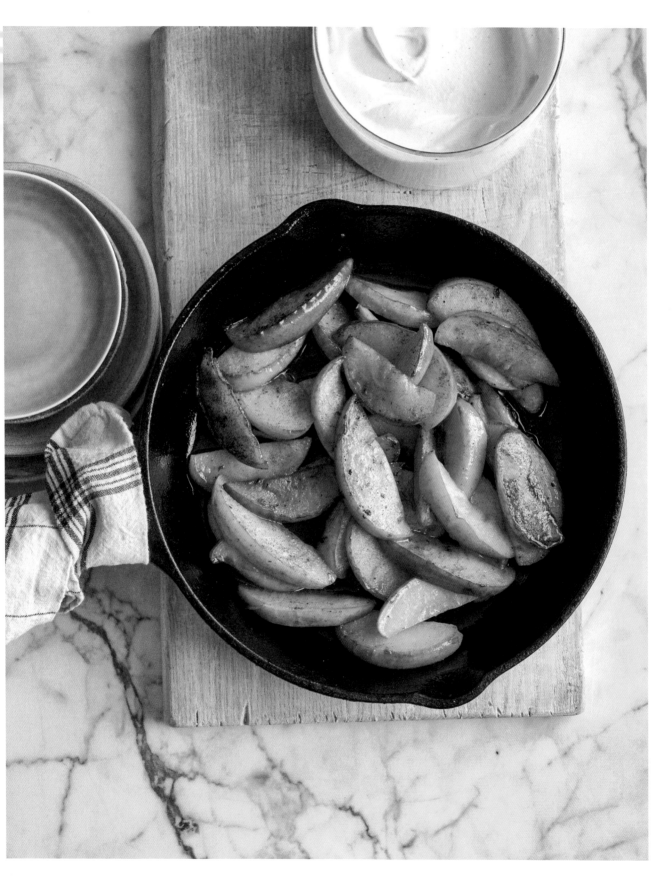

Mrs Adam's Rhubarb & Apple Crumble

I can't bear to completely turn my back on traditional puddings or watch my rhubarb patch turn to compost, so I like to find ways to eat it without the usual amounts of sugar. Our friend Sian Adams follows a low-carb diet and was looking for dessert inspiration. Glancing out of the kitchen window, she noticed some apples that had dropped onto her rhubarb patch from her neighbour's garden; of course – the apples would sweeten the sour stalks of rhubarb! This is lovely served with vanilla ice cream (see opposite), Greek yogurt, or double cream.

Preheat the oven to 200°C/fan 180°C/gas mark 6.

Put all the filling ingredients into a medium saucepan and simmer over a medium heat for 10 minutes, or until the fruit has softened.

Meanwhile, make the crumble. Add the butter and ground almonds to a mixing bowl and rub them together with your fingertips until they resemble breadcrumbs. Add the remaining ingredients and mix them through, breaking up the flaked almonds a little. Set aside.

Put the filling into an ovenproof dish measuring approx. 25 × 20 × 6cm (10 × 8 × 2½in) and cover with the crumble topping. Bake for 25 minutes, or until crisp and golden on top. Serve warm with a drizzle of vanilla oil, ice cream, Greek yogurt, or double cream.

SERVES 6

For the filling
4 long rhubarb stalks (approx.
   350g/12oz), roughly chopped
1 dessert apple, skin on, core
   removed, coarsely grated
thumb-sized piece of fresh ginger,
   peeled and finely grated
4 Medjool dates, stoned and finely
   chopped
100ml (3½fl oz) hot water

For the crumble
50g (2oz) butter, softened
150g (5oz) ground almonds
100g (3½oz) flaked almonds
½ teaspoon ground cinnamon
1 teaspoon vanilla powder or
   1½ teaspoons vanilla extract

Per serving 19g carbs,
10g protein, 30g fat, 8g fibre,
410kcal

Vanilla Ice Cream

After many trials, Stefano Borella – Head Chef of our cookery school – perfected this recipe for a creamy, intensely flavoured "iced cream", sweetened with dates and providing a base for many other flavours.

Heat the dates in 100ml (3½fl oz) of the cream in a cup in the microwave on full power for 1 minute or in a small pan over a medium heat until they soften. As soon as they are soft, pour the mixture into a sieve over a large bowl and use the back of a spoon to push it through. Discard the skin of the dates and add the remaining ingredients to the bowl. Mix thoroughly. Pour the mixture into a small container with a lid and put into the freezer. Stir every 30 minutes until set, or churn in an ice-cream machine.

To make the strawberry sauce, blend the strawberries and vanilla to a smooth purée. Pour it into a glass bowl and heat in the microwave or in a saucepan over a medium heat for a few minutes until the purée bubbles. It will thicken as it cooks and will be ready when it looks and smells like jam. Use straight away or cool and store in the fridge for up to 3 days, reheating as necessary.

Remove the ice cream from the freezer 15–20 minutes before serving. Serve in chilled glasses with the hot strawberry sauce or Vanilla Oil (page 63).

SERVES 4

1½ Medjool dates, stoned and finely chopped
300ml (10fl oz) double cream, coconut cream or full-fat Greek yogurt or a mixture of any
1/8 teaspoon xanthan gum
2 teaspoons vanilla extract

For the strawberry sauce
300g (10½oz) strawberries
1 teaspoon vanilla extract

Per serving of ice cream
8g carbs, 1.3g protein, 41g fat, 0.6g fibre, 403 kcal
Per serving of strawberry sauce
4.6g carbs, 0g protein, 0g fat, 2.8g fibre, 32kcal

Tahini Ice Cream

Our friend Anne Hudson came up with a genius idea for our tahini ice cream. To lighten the heaviness of the cream we have used Greek yogurt – and the tahini and yogurt are a marriage made in heaven.

Follow the recipe above to make the ice cream using half cream and half Greek yogurt. Add the tahini to the ice cream mix, pour the mixture into a small container with a lid and put into the freezer to set.

To make the hot chocolate sauce, heat the cream in a microwave or in a small pan over a medium heat until it just starts to bubble. Stir in the chocolate until it melts. Pour straight away over the ice cream in chilled glasses with the sesame seeds scattered over the top.

SERVES 4

2 tablespoons tahini
1 tablespoon toasted sesame seeds, to serve

For the hot chocolate sauce
50ml (2fl oz) single cream
25g (1oz) dark chocolate (85 per cent cocoa solids), finely chopped

Per serving of tahini ice cream
8g carbs, 3.9g protein, 47g fat, 1.6g fibre, 474kcal
Per serving of chocolate sauce
1.7g carbs, 1g protein, 5.7g fat, 0.7g fibre, 64kcal

Quick Whipped Cheesecake Shots

I have always been a sucker for the creamy acidity of a cheesecake, but since going low-carb they seem cloyingly sweet. I created this recipe so that we can indulge in my favourite dessert without worrying about our waistlines. Our friend Smithy came up with the idea of adding fresh ginger to the base – genius! Sometimes I leave out the base and serve the cream scattered with fresh blueberries, strawberries or slices of pear.

Preheat the oven to 200°C/fan 180°C/gas mark 6. Line a baking tray with baking parchment.

For the base, put the nuts onto the lined tray and toast in the oven for 8 minutes, or until lightly browned. Remove from the oven and set aside to cool while you make up the cream.

Mix the cheeses together with the vanilla and lemon zest. Taste and add more lemon or vanilla as necessary. Stir in the diced pear.

To finish the base, cut the date into small pieces and put into a cup with the boiling water. Mash it up with a fork and add it to a small food-processor, along with the toasted nuts, butter and ginger and whizz together to mix. If you don't have a food-processor, crush the nuts in a plastic bag with a rolling pin, grate the ginger and mix in a bowl with the other base ingredients.

Push the nutty mixture into the bottom of six small glasses. Divide the cream between them, allowing it to fall from the spoon (with the help of another spoon) into the centre of each glass so you don't smear the glass on the way in, then smooth the tops. They will keep like this for up to 3 days in the fridge without the berries. When you are ready to serve, top with the berries or pear slices and serve within 1 hour.

SERVES 6

For the base
100g (3½oz) hazelnuts, walnuts, pecans or almonds
1 Medjool date, stoned
2 tablespoons boiling water
10g (¼oz) butter
15g (½oz) fresh ginger, peeled or
1 teaspoon ground ginger

For the cream
180g (6½oz) cream cheese
250g (9oz) ricotta
2 teaspoons vanilla extract
zest of 1 lemon
100g (3½oz) ripe pears or pear quarters drained from a small can, finely diced

To serve
250g (9oz) berries or slices of pear

Per serving 9.7g carbs, 18g protein, 31g fat, 2.5g fibre, 390kcal

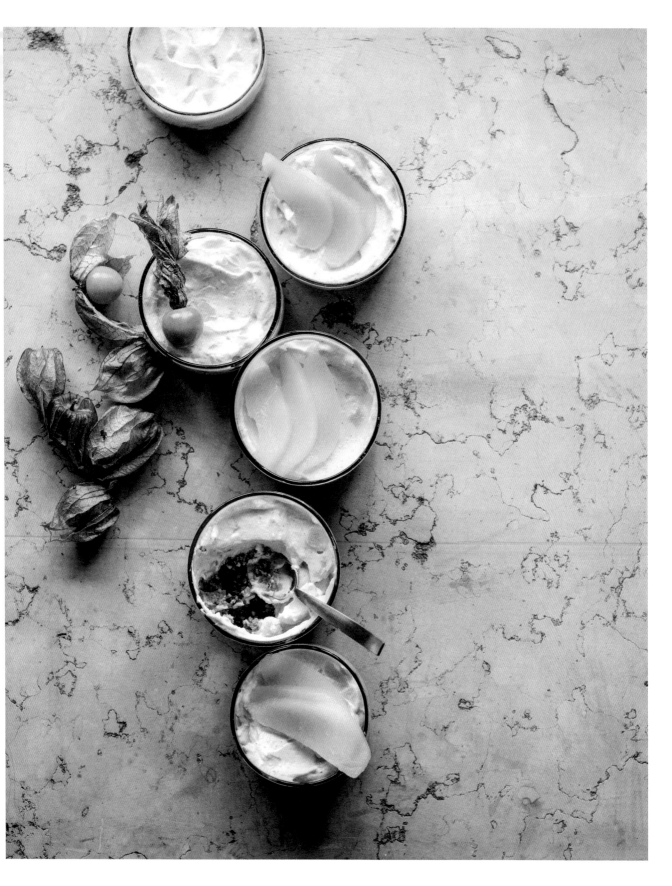

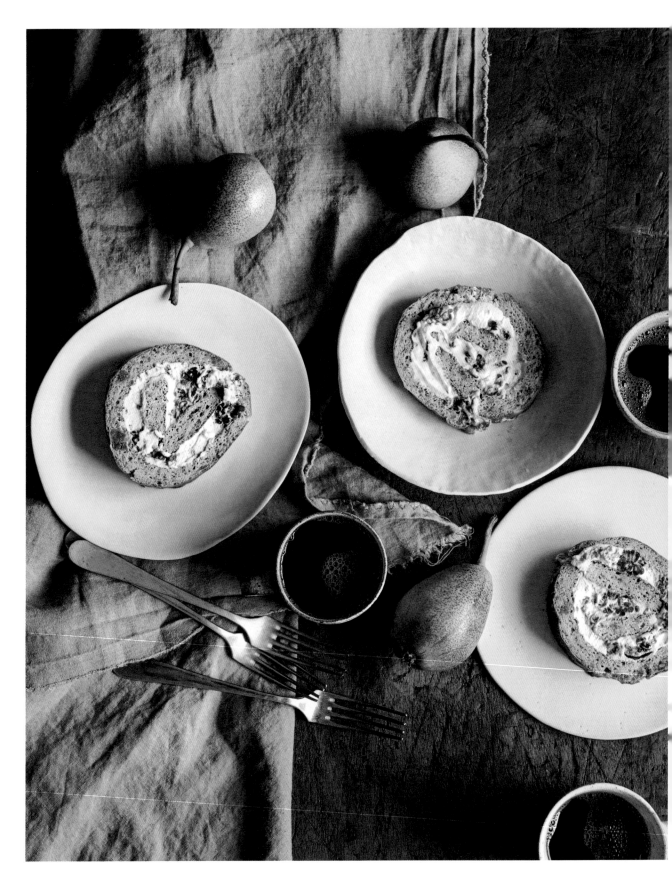

Hazelnut, Pear & Raspberry Roulade

This stunning dessert can be made with any ripe, seasonal low-carb fruit. We even found a cheat to get ripe fruit – use canned fruit and drain the fruit from the sweet juices to halve the carbs.

Preheat the oven to 200°C/fan 180°C/gas mark 6. Line two baking trays with baking parchment.

Put the hazelnuts onto one of the lined trays and roast for 10 minutes, or until golden brown. Remove from the oven and set aside to cool.

When the hazelnuts are cool, tip them into a food-processor using the baking parchment. Blitz until you have a sandy texture with some larger pieces to give a little crunch. Tip into a mixing bowl.

Add the pear to the bowl along with the egg yolks. Add the baking powder, vanilla and salt and stir through.

In a separate bowl, whisk the egg whites with an electric whisk until stiff peaks form. Add 2 tablespoons of the whisked egg whites to the nutty mixture and stir through with a large spatula.

Tip the remaining egg whites into the bowl and fold in gently. Spoon onto the remaining lined baking tray and spread out with a palette knife or flat-ended tool to a depth of 5mm (¼in). Bake for 10 minutes until the sponge is just set, firm and browned. Remove from the oven and turn upside down onto a clean tea towel. Remove the paper and roll the sponge into a spiral around the tea towel. Set aside to cool.

To make the filling, cut the dates into small pieces and put into a cup with the boiling water. Mash them with a fork and push through a sieve into a large mixing bowl. Add the cream, vanilla extract and lemon zest and whip until thickened with a balloon whisk or electric mixer. Stir in the fruit.

Unwind the hazelnut sponge leaving it on the tea towel. Spread the filling over it using a palette knife, leaving a clean border along the long edges of about 5cm (2in). Use the tea towel to help roll up the sponge around the cream filling creating a spiral. It should overlap slightly to seal in the filling. Arrange the roulade on a serving platter with the seam underneath. Put into the fridge to chill for a minimum of an hour and up to a day before serving.

MAKES 1 ROULADE/SERVES 8

200g (7oz) hazelnuts, skinned
1 ripe pear (approx. 125g/4½oz), peeled, cored and coarsely grated
4 eggs, separated
1 heaped teaspoon baking powder
2 teaspoons vanilla extract
pinch of salt

For the filling

2 Medjool dates, stoned
2 tablespoons boiling water
400ml (14fl oz) whipping cream
2 teaspoons vanilla extract
finely grated zest of 1 lemon
200g (7oz) raspberries or halved strawberries, or 250g (9oz) ripe or canned and drained pears, diced

Per serving 10g carbs, 9.3g protein, 39g fat, 4.7g fibre, 437kcal

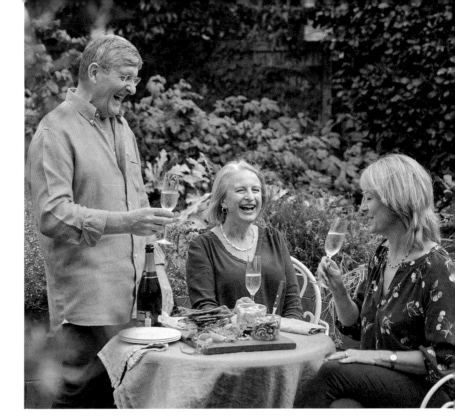

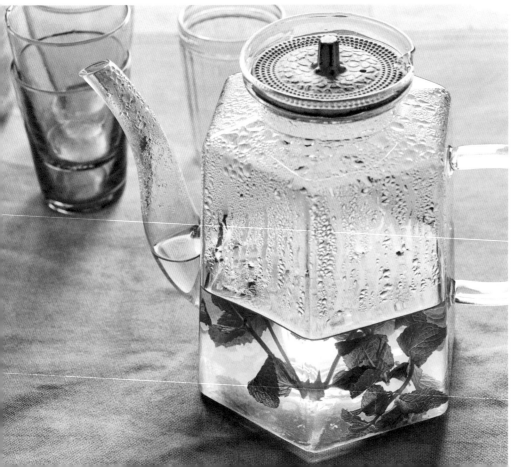

DRINKS

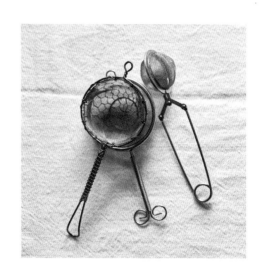

Drinks can help keep you going until the next meal when you feel hungry or tired. However, it is all too easy to reach for a cold can of fizz, fruit juice, sweet tea or cool beer without realizing the sugar content. Low-sugar versions often contain colouring, preservatives and artificial sweeteners – see page 38 for our reasons not to drink them. In this chapter, we give you some ideas that will comfort and nourish you and that are natural and not loaded with sugar.

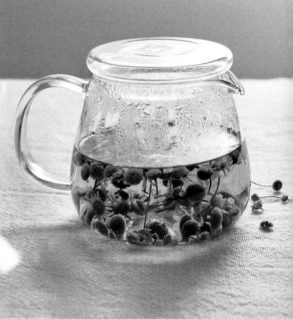

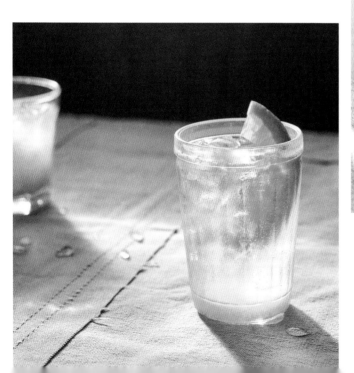

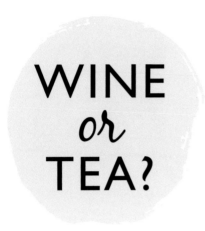

WINE
or
TEA?

I find being low-carb means my tolerance to alcohol has dropped; two small glasses of wine are now all my head and body can cope with. This means being more diligent when I am out, but it is better for my health and my pocket.

When people yearn for a drink it is often because they are craving sugar to wake them up. Instead of reaching for the wine, have a lovely low-carb drink in a wine glass and see how you feel before you reach for the corkscrew – see our suggestions on the following pages. Try distraction techniques – make a cup of one of the interesting teas below. I love the spiced ginger tea on my non-drinking nights. It gives a kick of heat in the same way alcohol does. The cravings for alcohol, like sugar or any carbs, pass with time so hang on in there. It is too easy for people to down half a bottle of wine a night and wonder why they have no energy or can't lose weight.

Coffee & tea

Redbush and herbal teas have no carbs and are naturally caffeine-free. Green tea enthusiasts insist that it helps with weight loss. It does have some medicinal properties so give it a try.

Fresh herbs from your garden also make excellent tea:

MINT TEA:
Put a large handful of mint leaves into a teapot and leave to stand for 5 minutes. Pour out and enjoy the cooling comfort of fresh mint tea.

BAY, ROSEMARY AND FENNEL TEA
Add a sprig of one or all of these herbs to a mug or teapot as above.

GINGER TEA
Add a couple of slices of fresh, peeled (no need to peel it if it is organic) ginger to boiling water.

COFFEE
The best way to drink coffee for weight-loss is black. But if you prefer it white then it is worth noting 1 Americano with 2 teaspoons double cream has 0g carbs while 1 Americano with 30ml whole milk has 1.3g carbs, so cream is back on the menu for low-carbers.

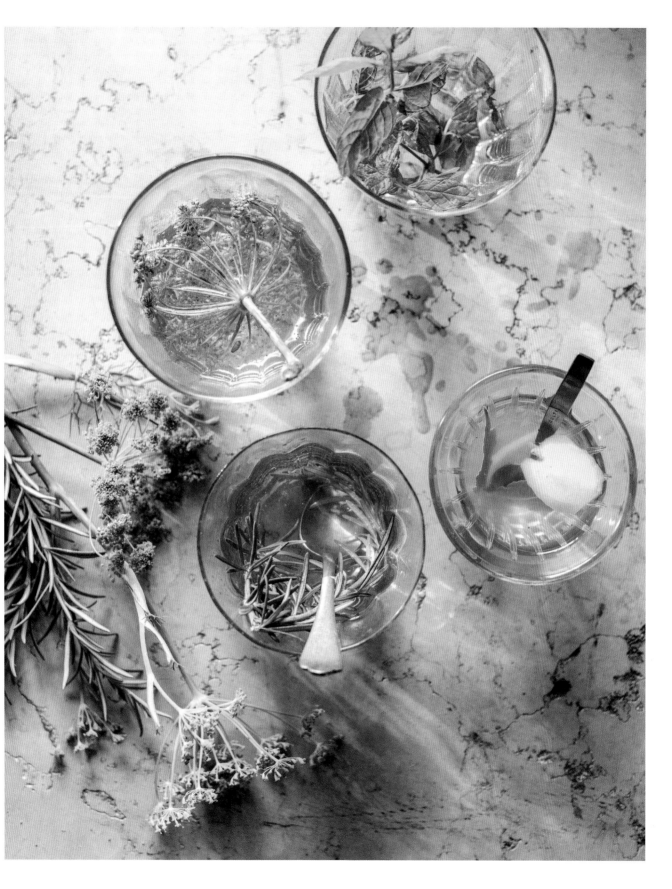

Lime Soda

While travelling around India, we loved to order this refreshing drink. Now we make it at home in large wine glasses with plenty of ice. A long slice of cucumber is also good dropped in. Add 5oml (2fl oz) of gin, rum or vodka to the mix for lime soda with a kick.

Pour the lime juice into a glass over a handful of ice (if using), add a pinch of salt and top up with soda water. Wipe the lime wedge around the rim of the glass and drop it inside before serving.

SERVES 1

1 tablespoon fresh lime juice
salt
1 small bottle soda water or 250ml
 (9fl oz) sparkling water
1 lime wedge

Per serving with gin *0g carbs, 0g protein, 0g fat, 0g fibre, 117kcal*

Angostura Orange

Bright and punchy with the tiniest hint of alcohol in the Angostura, this is a grown-up soft drink with no added sugar. It makes a good lunchtime drink and, while everyone else knocks back the alcohol, you can sip this with a smug smile as you won't be falling asleep in the afternoon.

Put the orange slice, juice and Angostura bitters into a large glass with a few ice cubes. Top up with soda water and serve straight away.

SERVES 1

1 orange slice
1 tablespoon freshly squeezed orange
 juice
few drops of Angostura bitters
a few ice cubes
1 small bottle soda water or 250ml
 (9fl oz) sparkling water

Per serving *8g carbs, 0g protein, 0g fat, 0g fibre, 9kcal*

Behind the Bar

This is basically all the fruit and herbs that you see behind a bar mixed with sparkling water. I ask our bartenders to put a slice of lime, orange, lemon and cucumber and a sprig of mint into a large glass and top up with sparkling water and ice. It is delicious and is usually readily available at good bars.

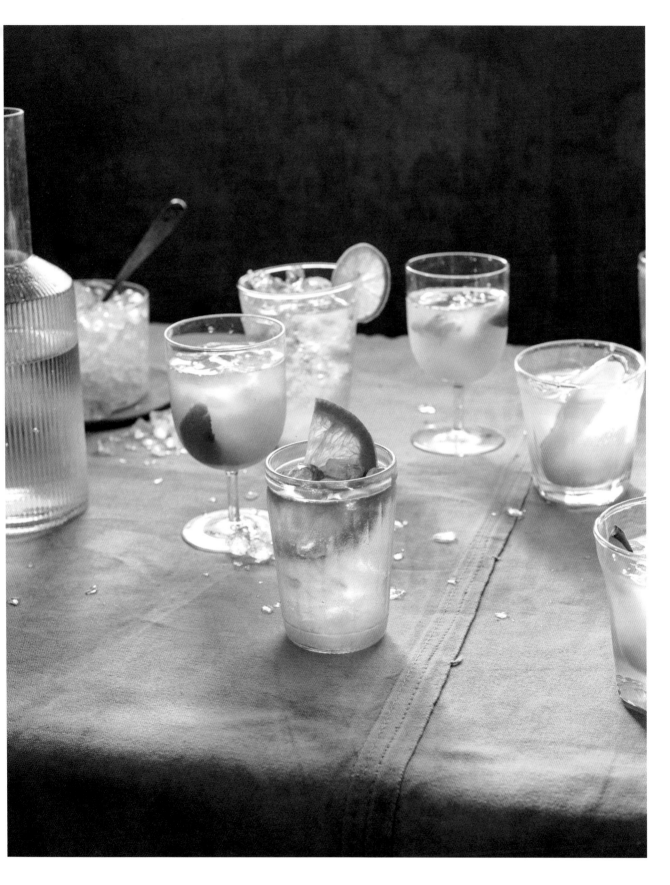

Ginger Juice and A Ginger, Lime & Mint Sparkler

This is my go-to summer drink. I love it so much I take a small bottle of ginger juice out with me as I know it isn't commercially available (yet!). It is so much better than most soft drinks that are full of sugar or sweeteners. Although you can buy small bottles of "ginger shots" they are mainly apple juice which is very high in sugar. It is great for no-booze nights as it still has a kick from the heat of the ginger rather than from alcohol.

To make the ginger juice, whizz the ginger and water together in a blender and then strain the juice through a fine sieve into a jar. Discard the fibrous ginger left in the sieve. Put the lid on the jar and store in the fridge until needed. It will keep for up to a week.

To drink, mix 2 tablespoons of the ginger juice with still or sparkling water in a long glass.

For a **Ginger, Lime & Mint Sparkler**, muddle a lime wedge and 6 mint leaves together in a glass to release the aromatics from them. Add a handful of ice and 2 tablespoons of ginger juice, followed by 250ml sparkling water. Add more lime or ginger to taste. Serve straight away. Add 50ml white or dark rum to make a cocktail.

MAKES APPROX. 200ML (7FL OZ), enough for 6 long sparkling ginger drinks

100g (3½oz) fresh ginger, peeled
150ml (5fl oz) still or sparkling water, to serve

Per serving *1.3g carbs, 0g protein, 0g fat, 0g fibre, 8kcal*

Quick Hot Chocolate

Raw cacao powder is high in iron, potassium, magnesium and fibre. It is also rich in antioxidant flavonoids called flavanols which may increase brain function. Flavanols are normally stripped away when chocolate is made and most good effects would be negated by the use of sugar in the processing. Raw cacao, on the other hand, retains more flavanols. Cinnamon helps to slow down the insulin spike caused by sweet foods and the vanilla extract suggests a bit of sweetness to satisfy that sweet tooth.

Heat the almond milk in a saucepan over a low heat and stir in the cacao powder and vanilla extract. Pour into a mug, dust with cinnamon and serve.

SERVES 1

1 mug of almond milk
2 heaped teaspoons raw cacao powder
a few drops of vanilla extract, added to taste
¼ teaspoon ground cinnamon

Per serving *4g carbs, 5.5g protein, 6.1g fat, 4.7g fibre, 102kcal*

Instant Cardamom & Turmeric Chai

I asked our neighbour Susie Batra to show me her version of India's famous health-giving chai or "golden milk". She showed me this recipe and called it her "inflammation buster" – I liked that! Shop-bought varieties of chai are usually very expensive or have powdered milk or sweeteners added. I make the mixture up in batches so that it is easy for me to take a little powder, pour on hot water and add a dash of milk. The ghee can be added for extra satiety.

To make the chai powder, mix together all the dry ingredients and store in a small jar.

When ready to drink, put ½ teaspoon of the chai powder in a mug and fill almost full with boiling water. Top up with cow's milk or unsweetened nut or coconut milk and 1 teaspoon of ghee (if using). Add the fresh ginger slices (if using) to serve.

SERVES APPROX. 12

2 teaspoons ground cardamom
1½ teaspoons ground turmeric
½ teaspoon freshly ground black
   pepper, to taste
1 teaspoon ground cinnamon
1 teaspoon ground ginger
2 thin slices fresh ginger, peeled, per
   mug, to serve (optional)
1 teaspoon of ghee per mug, to serve
   (optional)

Per serving with ghee and cow's milk *0.6g carbs, 0g protein, 0.6g fat, 0g fibre, 9kcal*

Chai Tea

This is from our Kuwaiti friend Amal. She bought me a teapot that sits over a candle to keep the tea piping hot – it's a beautiful sight and keeps me going in winter when I'm at my desk. The tea is gently heated with cream and infused with spices before straining into the pot.
Add all the ingredients, except the ginger, to a small pan. Bring to the boil, reduce the heat and simmer gently for 5–10 minutes, or until the chai starts to foam and bubble. Strain into a warm teapot, add the ginger (if using) and serve.

SERVES 4

650ml (23fl oz) hot water
2 black tea bags
4 cardamom pods, lightly crushed
4 cloves
pinch of saffron threads (optional)
½ teaspoon ground cinnamon
8cm (3¼in) piece of cinnamon stick
50ml (2fl oz) double cream
few slices of fresh ginger, peeled
   (optional)

Per serving *0.5g carbs, 0g protein, 6.5g fat, 0g fibre, 62kcal*

Appendix: Nutrient tables

These tables are to help familiarise you with the carbohydrate levels of foods, together with their fat, protein and fibre content. Mostly these are foods that you are encouraged to eat; those in bold are either less desirable versus others in the category (eg breaded chicken) or are high in absolute levels of carbs (eg dates).

Each recipe in this book has the nutrient levels already calculated for you. Another source of info is an app or book such as *Carbs & Cals*. Please be aware that there is some discrepancy between different sources of nutrient information so try to choose one method for tracking and stick to it or things can get confusing!

PROTEIN FOODS – Meat

	Weight	Cals	Fat	Carbs	Fibre	Protein
Chicken, breast	120g	174	2	0	0	38
Chicken, thigh	120g	193	7	0	0	33
Turkey breast	120g	186	2	0	0	42
Turkey, dark meat	120g	213	8	0	0	35
Venison	120g	198	3	0	0	43
Duck	120g	234	12	0	0	30
Lamb leg	120g	290	16	0	0	36
Lamb shoulder	120g	282	16	0	0	34
Pork chop	120g	221	8	0	0	38
Pork scratchings	30g	182	14	0	0	14
Pork roast	120g	258	12	0	0	37
Sausages 97% meat (2)	112g	301	24	2	1	19
Bacon (2 rashers)	60g	172	13	0	0	14
Sirloin steak	200g	425	25	0	0	50
Roast beef	120g	293	15	0	0	39
Breaded chicken	**120g**	**281**	**14**	**17**	**1**	**21**

PROTEIN FOODS – Eggs & dairy

	Weight	Cals	Fat	Carbs	Fibre	Protein
Eggs (one)	54g	97	7	0	0	8
Full-fat Greek yogurt	100g	117	7	3.8	0	9.8
Low-fat fruit yogurt	**100g**	**82**	**1**	**13**	**0**	**4**
Cheddar	75g	311	26	0	0	19
Feta	75g	186	15	1	0	11
Roquefort	75g	280	25	0	0	14
Milk (full fat)	200ml	126	7	9	0	7
Milk (semi-skimmed)	200ml	94	3	9	0	7
Milk (skimmed)	200ml	70	1	9	0	7
Double cream	30ml	149	16	0	0	0

PROTEIN FOODS – Seafood

	Weight	Cals	Fat	Carbs	Fibre	Protein
Salmon	120g	245	15	0	0	28
Mackerel	120g	339	27	0	0	24
Prawns, peeled, frozen	120g	86	0.2	0	0	19
Sardines, tinned	85g	187	12	0	0	20
Cod in breadcrumbs, baked	120g	242	14	12	1	17

PROTEIN – Vegetarian

	Weight	Cals	Fat	Carbs	Fibre	Protein
Puy lentils, half pack	**125g**	**180**	**2**	**24**	**8**	**12**
Chickpeas, half pack	115g	130	3	14	10	8

STARCHY FOODS – Vegetables

	Weight	Cals	Fat	Carbs	Fibre	Protein
Beetroot	100g	41	0	7	2	2
Butternut squash	100g	42	0	8	2	1
Carrots	100g	44	0	8	4	0
Celeriac	100g	26	0	2	4	1
Parsnip	100g	73	1	12	5	2
Potato (peeled)	200g	168	0	36	4	4
Pumpkin	100g	15	0	2	1	1
Swede	100g	30	0	5	2	1
Sweet potato	**100g**	**91**	**0**	**20**	**2**	**1**
Sweetcorn	80g	55	2	6	3	2
Turnip	100g	30	0	5	2	1

STARCHY FOODS – Grains & seeds

	Weight	Cals	Fat	Carbs	Fibre	Protein
Brown bread (1 slice)	40g	86	1	15	2	4
Brown rice	50g	177	1	35	3	5
Chapati	55g	186	7	24	3	5
Oats	35g	137	3	22	3	4
Pasta	75g	261	2	51	4	9
Quinoa	50g	160	3	26	4	7
Rye bread (1 slice)	72g	163	1	30	3	6
White bread (1 slice)	40g	89	1	17	1	4
White rice	50g	171	1	37	1	4

SUPERVEG

	Weight	Cals	Fat	Carbs	Fibre	Protein
Asparagus	80g	23	0	2	1	2
Aubergine	80g	16	0	2	2	1
Avocado, half	80g	158	16	2	3	2
Broccoli	80g	35	0	3	3	3
Brussel sprouts	80g	41	1	3	3	3
Cabbage	80g	25	0	4	2	1
Cauliflower	80g	33	0	6	1	2
Celery	80g	10	0	2	1	0
Courgettes	80g	18	0	1	2	1
Cucumber	80g	13	0	1	1	1
Fennel	80g	16	0	1	3	1
Garlic	10g	11	0	2	0	1
Green beans	80g	25	0	2	3	2
Kale	80g	33	1	1	3	3
Lettuce	60g	8	0	1	1	1
Leeks	80g	22	0	2	2	1
Mooli	80g	13	0	2	0	1
Mushrooms	80g	17	0	2	1	2
Olives	15g	17	2	0	1	0
Onions	50g	21	0	4	1	1
Peas	80g	62	1	8	4	4
Peppers	60g	16	0	3	1	0
Rocket	60g	13	0	0	1	2
Spinach	60g	11	0	0	1	2
Tomatoes	60g	13	0	2	1	0
Watercress	60g	17	1	0	2	2

FRUIT

	Weight	Cals	Fat	Carbs	Fibre	Protein
Apples	130g	56	0	13	1	0
Apricot	55g	17	0	4	1	1
Apricot, dried (4)	32g	81	0	16	7	2
Banana	130g	69	0	17	1	1
Blackberries	80g	20	0	4	3	1
Blueberries	80g	32	0	7	2	1
Cherries	100g	48	0	12	1	1
Dates (4)	30g	81	0	20	2	1
Grapefruit	114g	2	0	1	0	0
Honeydew Melon	160g	45	0	11	2	2
Kiwi	55g	27	0	6	1	1
Mango	120g	68	0	17	5	1
Nectarine	140g	56	0	13	3	1
Orange	140g	38	0	8	1	1
Papaya	80g	29	0	7	2	0
Peach	140g	46	0	11	3	1
Pineapple	150g	75	0	15	3	0
Plum	110g	40	0	10	2	1
Pomegranate	80g	67	1	13	2	1
Raspberries	80g	20	0	4	2	1
Strawberries	140g	42	0	8	6	1
Sultanas	30g	83	0	21	1	1

OILS – Oil & fats

	Weight	Cals	Fat	Carbs	Fibre	Protein
Butter	10g	75	8	0	0	0
Coconut oil	10g	90	10	0	0	0
Olive oil	10g	90	10	0	0	0

OILS – Nuts & seeds

	Weight	Cals	Fat	Carbs	Fibre	Protein
Almond	30g	185	16	2	5	6
Brazil	30g	212	20	1	2	5
Cashew	30g	178	14	5	1	6
Coconut, desiccated	30g	196	19	2	6	2
Flax seed	15g	85	7	0	4	3
Hazelnut	30g	204	19	2	3	5
Peanut	30g	181	16	2	2	8
Pumpkin seed	15g	89	7	2	1	4
Sesame seed	15g	95	9	0	1	3
Sunflower seed	15g	90	7	3	1	3
Walnut	30g	213	21	1	2	5

Index

Resources & References

Primarily we used **www.nutritics.com** for the nutritional analysis.

Diabetes.co.uk, the global diabetes community.

www.lowcarbprogram.com is a digital program that redefines metabolic health.

Carbs & Cals produce carb and calorie counter books and apps.

Freestyle Libre makes instant glucose monitoring systems and can be found at **www.freestylelibre.co.uk.**

The Public Health Collaboration is a charity dedicated to informing and implementing decisions for better public health. Find out more at **www.phcuk.org.**

See **www.westonaprice.org** for information nutrition and health.

See **www.dietdoctor.com** for information on low-carb diets

For a list of scientific references please go to **www.inspirednutrition.co.uk**

Acknowledgements

Giancarlo, Jenny and I were delighted to work with Dr David Unwin and Dr Jen Unwin on this project. Their knowledge, experience and help were invaluable. We wish it to be known that they have received no fee for their participation in this book. Instead we made a donation to the Public Health Collaboration to further the work to further their work spreading the real food message.

A huge thank you to everyone who suggested and tested recipes with me for this book: Anne Hudson, Karin Piper, Nina Power, Sohini Basu, Pratima Basu, Amal Al Alquatani, Stefano Borella, Brian McLeod, Louli Ford, Carly Roberts, Philip Beresford, Anita Zgrablic, Susie Batra and Claire "Smithy" Smith. Karen Courtney, Lorna Smalley and Jim Davies for their encouragement and support. Vicky Orchard, editor. Susan Bell for the stunning photography. Susie, Claudia and Sami for the beautiful food and prop styling. Tina Smith for the design of the book. Emily Noto for the production.

And last but definitely not least thank you to our boys Giorgio and Flavio for their endless help in cooking, tasting good (and bad!) recipes, constant washing and drying up. And sorry for the repetitive lectures about not eating sugar and generally my lack of attention for the past two years when you tried to tell me about particle physics while I was finishing the book.

Find Katie and Giancarlo at **www.caldesi.com**, on Instagram and Twitter **@katiecaldesi**, Facebook under Caldesi Italian Restaurants. Dr David Unwin **@lowcarbGP**, Dr Jen Unwin **@jen_unwin** and/or **@realfoodrocksUK**, Jenny Phillips on twitter **@jennynutrition** and **www.inspirednutrition.co.uk**

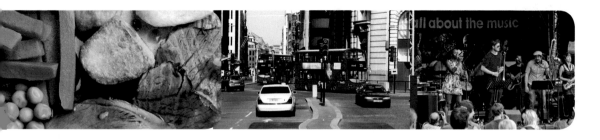

CONTENTS

• •

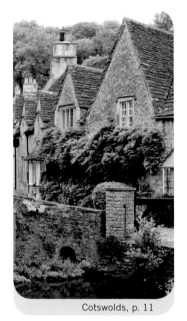

Cotswolds, p. 11

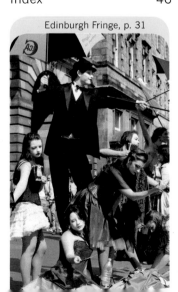

Edinburgh Fringe, p. 31

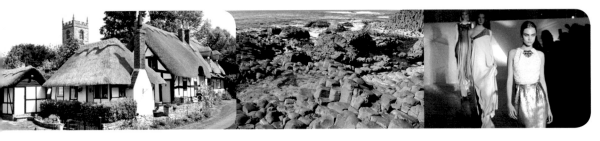

WHAT'S HOT: UK

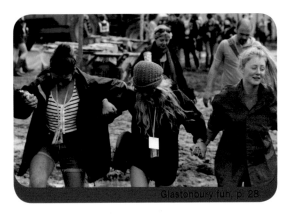

Glastonbury fun, p. 28

There is always something to see or do in the UK – whether you want to hike through misty mountains, listen to live music at a festival, watch some of the world's top football teams, tuck into a legendary Cornish pasty or shop at some of the best street markets around.

1. TAKE A BORIS BIKE TOUR OF LONDON p.12

Named after London's eccentric mayor, Boris Johnson, (although they were the previous mayor's idea!) the simple blue bikes are everywhere and are a great way to see the city.

2. HUNT FOR VINTAGE THREADS AT OLD SPITALFIELDS p.14

London is jammed with street markets; this is a great one for vintage clothes, one-off pieces by new designers and ethnic fabrics.

3. EAT A FULL ENGLISH p.18

Few people eat this traditional breakfast every day, but it's a shame not to give it a try. Just don't plan to do anything energetic afterwards!

4. WATCH THE BOAT RACE p.22

One of the oldest and most famous rowing races in the world, the Boat Race was first held in 1829. You can watch free from the banks of the River Thames, or crowd onto Hammersmith Bridge to watch the crews from above. It's also shown live on TV.

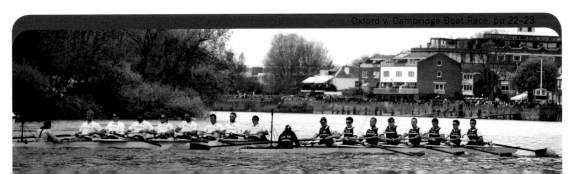

Oxford v. Cambridge Boat Race, pp 22–23

5. GET MUDDY AT GLASTONBURY p.28

The UK's biggest and most famous music festival seems to get more than its fair share of rain. It's still fun – but don't forget your wellies.

6. SPEND A WEEKEND IN A TENT p.34

Camping is a great way to experience the UK countryside. In fact, you don't need a tent: you can camp in teepees, treehouses, yurts and all kinds of other oddball shelters.

7. GET ALL STEAMED UP IN DORSET p.36

Every August, steam-powered engines, tractors and other vehicles from around the country converge on north Dorset for the Great Dorset Steam Fair.

8. WATCH THE SUN SET AT CALLANISH p.38

This ancient stone circle on an isolated Scottish island is 4,500 years old – and standing there alone at sunset is as spooky now as it must have been then.

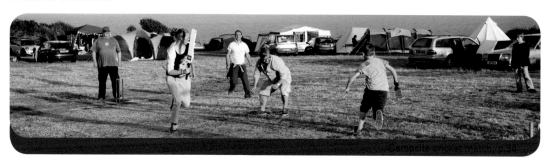
Campsite cricket match, p.32

PUBLIC HOLIDAYS

The UK has national holidays throughout the year; not all are held throughout the UK:

1 January	New Year's Day
2 January	(only in Scotland)
13 March	St Patrick's Day (Northern Ireland only)
Date changes:	Good Friday
Date changes: (England, Northern Ireland, Wales)	Easter Monday
First Monday in May	May Day
Last Monday in May	Spring Holiday
12 July	Orangemen's Day (Northern Ireland)
First Monday in August	Summer Holiday (Scotland)
Last Monday in August	Summer Holiday (England, Northern Ireland, Wales)
30 November	St Andrew's Day (Scotland only)
25 December	Christmas Day
26 December	Boxing Day

INTRODUCING THE UK

UK FACTS AND STATS

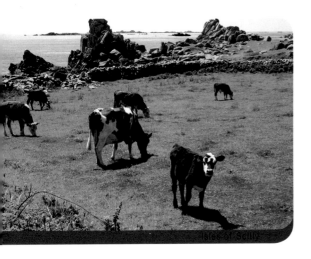
Isles of Scilly

The United Kingdom is not very big. In fact, there are 11 US states that are bigger!* But the UK packs a lot into a small space: it contains mountains, ancient monuments, beautiful islands, countryside peppered with thatched cottages and one of the world's most famous cities – London.

*It's smaller than Michigan (no. 11), but bigger than Minnesota (no. 12).

LANDSCAPE

The UK's landscape is mostly hilly. There is flatter land to the south and east, while North Wales and Scotland are mountainous. Landscape highlights to look out for include:

- The UK's tallest mountains in the Highlands of Scotland

- Hills topped with ancient standing stones on the moors of the southwest

- Sandy bays and towering cliffs on the Gower Peninsula, in Wales

- The Giant's Causeway, the remains of an ancient volcanic eruption in Northern Ireland

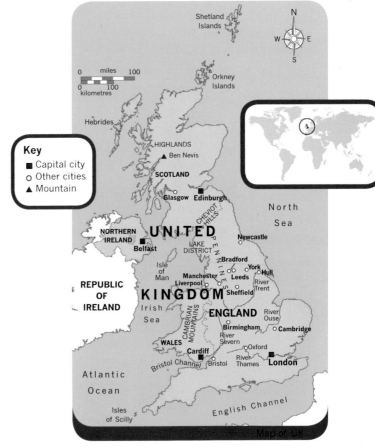

Key
- ■ Capital city
- ○ Other cities
- ▲ Mountain

Shetland Islands

Orkney Islands

Hebrides

HIGHLANDS
▲ Ben Nevis

SCOTLAND

Glasgow Edinburgh

NORTHERN IRELAND
Belfast

UNITED

LAKE DISTRICT

Newcastle

North Sea

CHEVIOT HILLS

PENNINES

Bradford

Isle of Man

Manchester Leeds

York

Hull

Liverpool

Sheffield

River Trent

REPUBLIC OF IRELAND

Irish Sea

KINGDOM

ENGLAND

River Ouse

CAMBRIAN MOUNTAINS

Birmingham

Cambridge

WALES

River Severn

Oxford

Cardiff

Bristol Channel Bristol

River Thames

London

Atlantic Ocean

Isles of Scilly

English Channel

Map of UK

CLIMATE

During winter, the UK's climate is cold enough for everyone to need coats, hats and gloves. In summer on some days, it is warm enough for swimming in the sea (tough people swim in the sea the rest of the year too). Throughout the year, temperatures are likely to be colder further north. Rainclouds can sweep in from the Atlantic Ocean at any time of year, but especially in winter.

WHAT IS THE UNITED KINGDOM?

Four areas make up the United Kingdom:

1. England, Scotland and Wales – occupy the island of Great Britain.

2. Northern Ireland – occupies the northeast part of the island of Ireland.

Confusingly, all citizens – even those from Northern Ireland – are commonly known as 'British' people.

FACT FILE ONE

CAPITAL CITY: London

AREA: 241,930km² of land area, plus 1,680 km² of sea area

HIGHEST MOUNTAIN: Ben Nevis, Scotland (1,343 m)

LOWEST POINT: The Fens (-4 m)

LONGEST RIVER: Severn (354 km)

BORDERS: Northern Ireland borders the Republic of Ireland

NATURAL HAZARDS: flooding, winter storms, blizzards

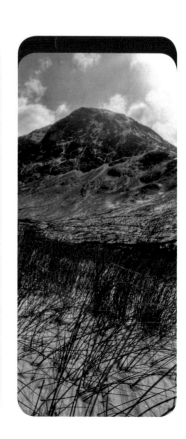

PEOPLE

The UK is a country of immigrants. In ancient times, Roman, Saxon and Norman invaders settled here, and immigrants have been arriving ever since. Recently, more peaceful settlers have come from South Asia, the Caribbean, Eastern Europe, Africa and many other parts of the world. Walk along a busy city street and you can hear the UK's diversity: Polish, Punjabi, Afghan, Australian, Cantonese, Czech, Slovak, Sinhalese and many other languages and accents.

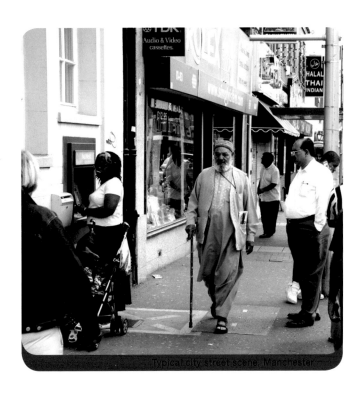
Typical city street scene, Manchester

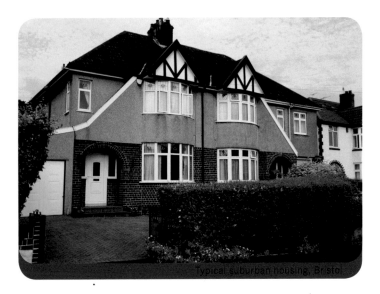
Typical suburban housing, Bristol

URBAN LIFE

Nearly all of the UK's people live in towns or cities. In city centres, most people live in a flat. Suburbs, where houses are more common, surround most cities. British homes are small compared to some other wealthy countries: on average, US and Australian homes are three times the size, and French homes are 50% bigger.

RURAL LIFE

Only one in 10 people lives in the countryside. Life in the countryside is more expensive than in towns and cities, because of transport and housing costs. Houses in pretty areas such as the Cotswolds are often bought as holiday homes. Many are empty outside the holiday season, giving some villages a ghost-town vibe.

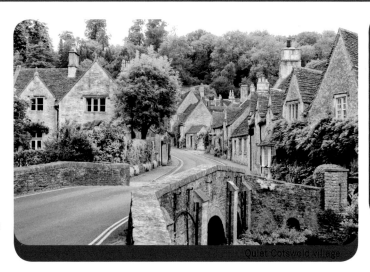
Quiet Cotswold village

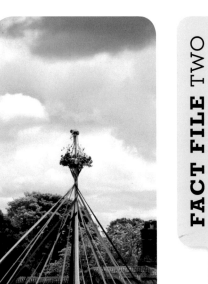
Village maypole dancing

FACT FILE TWO

POPULATION: 63 million

CITIES OF OVER 1 MILLION PEOPLE: London (8.61 million), Birmingham (2.3 million), Manchester (2.25 million), Glasgow (1.17 million)

AGE STRUCTURE: 17.3% under 15 years old; 65.8% 15–64 years old; 16.9% over 64 years old

YOUTH UNEMPLOYMENT (15–24 year-olds): 18.9%

OBESITY: 22.7%

LANGUAGES: English (official language); Scots, Scottish Gaelic, Welsh, Irish and Cornish are official regional languages. After English, Polish and Punjabi are the next most common languages

RELIGIONS: Christians make up 71.6% of the UK population, Muslims 2.7%, Hindus 1%, other religions 1%

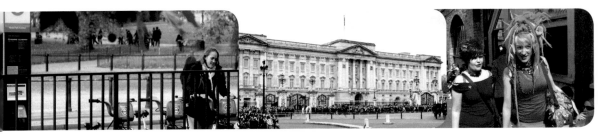

LONDON BIKE TOUR

L ondon is one of the world's most influential cities. It is a centre for fashion, art and music – and less interestingly, banking and finance. Ultra-modern buildings stand beside ancient ones from 500 years ago or more. Just wandering around the ancient streets gives you a buzz.

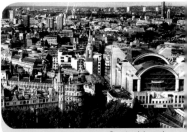

Central London

TAKE A KOOKY 'BORIS BIKE' TOUR

One of the best ways to see London is to pedal your way around on one of the city's 'Boris Bikes'. So, which places could you include on your kooky tour?

The smallest police station, Trafalgar Square, Central London (far right)

This police station is so small, even people who have been to Trafalgar Square probably won't have noticed it. It looks more like a telephone booth than a cop shop.

London catacombs, various locations

During the 1800s, London began to run out of places to put its dead. The answer was to create catacombs – passageways filled with tombs. One of the best is the half-underground one at Highgate Cemetery.

London's oldest inn, Wapping, East London

The Prospect of Whitby (below) has been an inn since the 1500s. It was once so popular with shady characters that it was called The Devil's Tavern. After a fire in the 1800s, the inn was renamed in the hope of attracting a better class of customer.

The Cathedral of Sewage, Newham, East London

'Cathedral of Sewage' is actually a nickname – this building's real name is Abbey Mills Pumping Station. It's one of the few parts of London's Victorian sewage system you can visit, though the tours only happen once a year (usually in May).

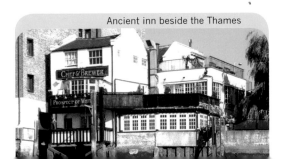

Ancient inn beside the Thames

BORIS BIKES

Boris Bikes are nicknamed after Mayor Boris Johnson. They can be hired at 'docking stations' (right) around London. You pay a small fee for access to the docking stations. After that, up to half an hour's bike use is free.

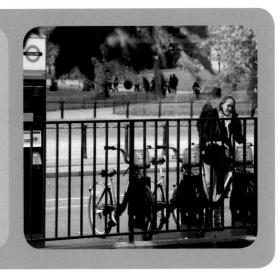

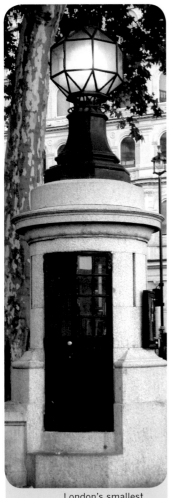

London's smallest police station

LONDON MYTHS

MYTH: There's a street lamp in Carting Lane that runs on sewer gas from the Savoy Hotel

Some London gas lamps once did run partly on sewer gas – but not any more. The one on Carting Lane is a replica of those old-style gas lamps.

MYTH: When the Union flag is flying over Buckingham Palace, the Queen is home

Actually, it means she's out. When Her Majesty is there, the Royal Standard will be flying.

MYTH: There are no 'Roads' in the City of London

People will often tell you that the City (the old Square Mile at the very heart of London) contains no routes called 'Road'. They're nearly correct – but since 1994, Goswell Road has technically been half in the City.

LONDON: FASHION CITY

Londra is the fashion capital of the UK, and one of the world's leading cities for clothing design. In fact, in 2012 London was voted the world's MOST fashionable city. Spend an hour or two in the coolest parts of town, and you're bound to see someone walk past wearing next year's look.

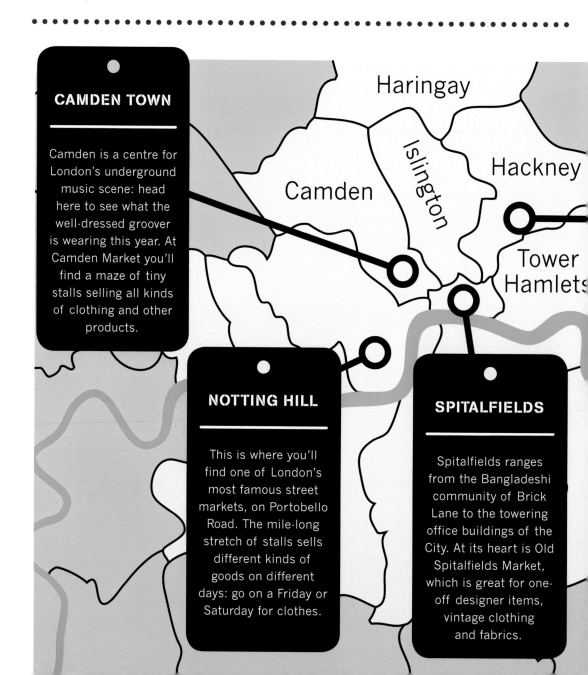

CAMDEN TOWN

Camden is a centre for London's underground music scene: head here to see what the well-dressed groover is wearing this year. At Camden Market you'll find a maze of tiny stalls selling all kinds of clothing and other products.

Haringay

Islington

Camden

Hackney

Tower Hamlets

NOTTING HILL

This is where you'll find one of London's most famous street markets, on Portobello Road. The mile-long stretch of stalls sells different kinds of goods on different days: go on a Friday or Saturday for clothes.

SPITALFIELDS

Spitalfields ranges from the Bangladeshi community of Brick Lane to the towering office buildings of the City. At its heart is Old Spitalfields Market, which is great for one-off designer items, vintage clothing and fabrics.

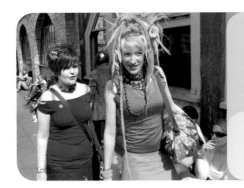

"You have a much better life if you wear impressive clothes."

— UK fashion designer Vivienne Westwood

HOXTON

The unofficial coolest neighbourhood in London, Hoxton is a great place for trend spotting. You'll laugh at the ridiculous fashions and haircuts – only to find yourself copying them in six months' time.

Greenwich

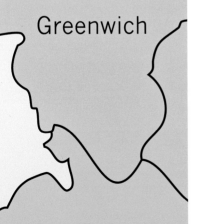

LONDON FASHION WEEK

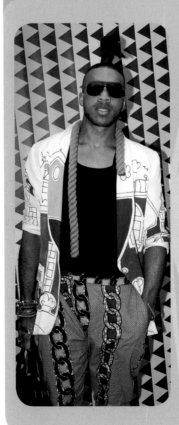

London Fashion Week is one of the world's biggest fashion events (the others are in New York, Paris and Milan). It is held twice a year, in February and September. Catwalk shows display designers' clothes for the next season.

It's basically impossible for ordinary people to get tickets, but some shows are now streamed live on the Internet.

BUCKINGHAM PALACE AND ROYAL BRITAIN

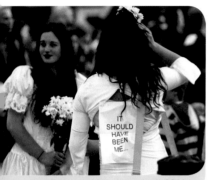
Royal wedding fever, April 2011

For the wedding of Prince William and Kate Middleton in 2011, and the 2012 Queen's Jubilee, everyone in the UK was given an extra day off work. They celebrated by wearing fancy dress, holding street parties and generally having a good time. No wonder the Royal Family is so popular!

BUCKINGHAM PALACE

You can't really visit London without a trip to Buckingham Palace. This has been the official home of the British monarch since 1837, when Queen Victoria saw its potential as a fixer-upper and moved in.

These days, millions of people visit Buckingham Palace each year. Mainly they have their photo taken outside, next to the unflinching, unsmiling Guardsmen. But the Queen's Gallery, where her art collection is displayed, is open to the public. It is also possible to visit the State Rooms during July and August.

> **"I am glad we have been bombed. Now I can look the East End in the face."**
>
> — Queen Elizabeth, wife of King George VI, after Buckingham Palace was bombed in 1940. The East End had already been hit by German bombers, and large areas destroyed.

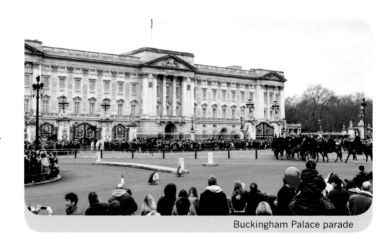
Buckingham Palace parade

A BRITISH STREET PARTY

How do you organise a British street party?
1. Ask the police for permission to close your street.
2. Set out long tables, chairs and Union Jack bunting.
3. Ask all your neighbours to bring food and drink: typically sandwiches, cakes, tea and squash.
4. Hope it doesn't rain!

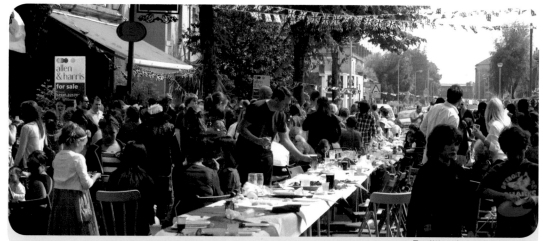

Traditional street party

OTHER ROYAL RESIDENCES

Buckingham Palace is not the Queen's only residence. Others include:

1. Sandringham House, Norfolk, England – Though it looks very old-fashioned now, Sandringham was once cutting edge. It had gas lamps, flushing toilets and even a shower when these things were very unusual. It is possible to visit the grounds and house at certain times of the year.

2. Balmoral Castle, Aberdeenshire, Scotland – Built for Queen Victoria in 1856, Balmoral's gardens are open to visitors from April to the end of July. It is also possible to visit the grand ballroom.

3. Windsor Castle, Berkshire, England – The original castle was built in the 11th century. It was used as a refuge for the Royal Family during air raids in the Second World War (1939–45) and survived a fire in 1992. The Queen likes to spend her weekends here.

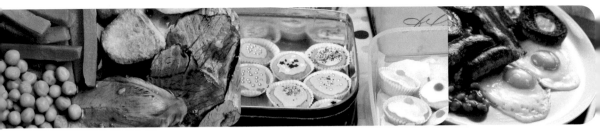

FOOD AND EATING

Most British people eat three meals a day: breakfast, lunch and dinner. Many also snack throughout the day – which might be why one in five of them are now dangerously overweight. People in the UK have an amazingly varied menu, which includes dishes from all round the world.

In the past, British food had a terrible reputation. People said that it was usually frozen, deep-fried or boiled to tastelessness – and they were mostly correct. These days, though, most British people prefer fresh ingredients cooked in a tasty, healthy way.

TYPICAL FOODS

These are a few typical UK dishes. Note that this isn't a typical day's eating – if you ate all these suggestions, you'd burst!

Breakfast (eaten between 07:30-09:30)

Most people have cereal or toast, with tea to drink. Every visitor to the UK should try the 'full English' breakfast once, though. This typically contains toast or fried bread, egg, bacon, sausage, mushrooms, baked beans, fried potato, black pudding and tomato. There are regional variations: full Scottish and Welsh breakfasts, and the 'Ulster fry'.

Lunch (eaten between 12:30-14:30)

Most adults eat a sandwich for lunch. Schools offer students a choice of food which usually includes salads, pasta and rice dishes. A weekend favourite is a Sunday roast, which is roast meat, roast potatoes, gravy and vegetables.

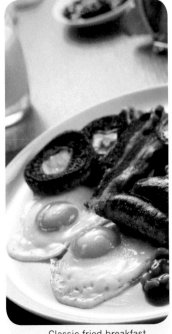

Classic fried breakfast

FOOD

Dinner, Tea or Supper
(eaten between 18:00-20:30)

Dinnertime really shows off the UK's multicultural history. In a typical week people might eat cottage pie, Thai curry, stir-fried meat and vegetables, spaghetti Bolognese, chicken curry and pizza.

"It takes some skill to spoil a breakfast – even the English can't do it."

— (American) economist JK Galbraith

WHAT'S IN A NAME?

In some areas of the UK, people call their meal in the middle of the day 'dinner', rather than 'lunch'. The evening meal is then known as 'tea'. Another term, 'supper', is used all over the UK. It may describe a light meal or snack that is eaten late at night – although for some it may be what they call the evening meal.

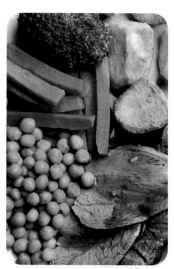

Sunday roast

THE UK'S TOP 10 MEALS

This list of the UK's 10 favourite family meals appeared in 2009:

1. Spaghetti Bolognese

2. Sunday roast

3. Chilli con carne

4. Lasagne

5. Cottage/shepherd's pie (cottage pie is made with beef, shepherd's pie with lamb)

6. Chinese stir fry

7. Beef stew

8. Macaroni cheese

9. Toad in the hole (sausages baked in batter)

10. Curry

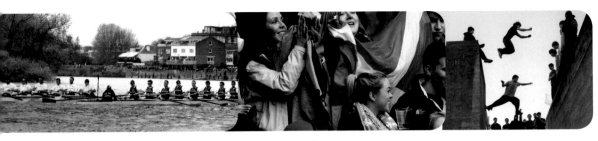

FOOTBALL AND THE FA CUP

Britain's favourite sport by far is football. The modern game was invented in Britain, then exported around the world. Sadly, the rest of the world soon got quite a lot better at it than the British. That hasn't stopped people loving football, though!

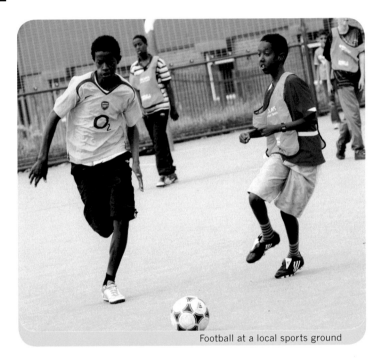

Football at a local sports ground

STREET FOOTBALL

You see street football being played everywhere in the UK. Any bit of waste ground, park or empty basketball court will probably have kids playing on it. Street football games normally use one 'goal' (which is often two piles of sweatshirts, or a space on a wall) and only need three players.

LEAGUE FOOTBALL

Most places in the UK have a proper 11-a-side football team, even small villages. As a result, on weekends during the season (August–May) you're never far from a game to watch. The sport is governed by the Football Association (FA), which organises leagues and other competitions.

"Some people believe football's a matter of life and death. I'm very disappointed with that attitude. I can assure you it's much more important than that."

— famous football manager Bill Shankly

THE FA CUP'S BIGGEST SHOCKS

1972: Hereford v. Newcastle

Newcastle are one of the country's top teams. Hereford don't even play in one of the top four divisions – but they still win 2–1. It is the biggest upset in FA Cup history.

1984: Bournemouth v. Manchester United

United are the UK's top team, and have won the Cup more times than anyone else. But they still get beaten 2–0 by Third Division (now called League One) Bournemouth.

The FA Cup

SPORT

THE FA CUP

The oldest football competition of all is the FA Cup. This is one of those sports events that even people who aren't interested in sport like to watch. Teams are drawn randomly to decide who plays one another. Some of the Cup's most exciting stories happen when a small team beats a bigger one. If you buy a ticket to one of the early rounds, you might even see a surprise result.

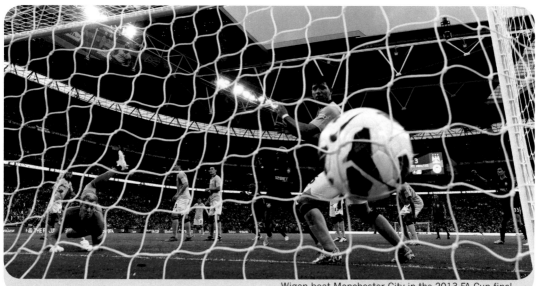

Wigan beat Manchester City in the 2013 FA Cup final

BIG UK EVENTS

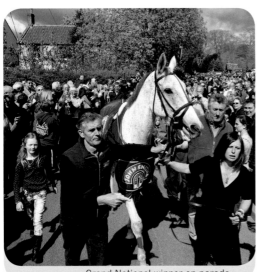

Grand National winner on parade

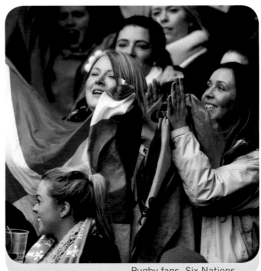

Rugby fans, Six Nations

Since London held the Olympic Games in 2012, the UK has been swept with enthusiasm for sport. The streets are full of people jogging, cycling or on their way to the gym, and it is difficult to get a ticket for any of the country's big sports events.

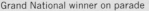

Boat Race crowds, Hammersmith Bridge

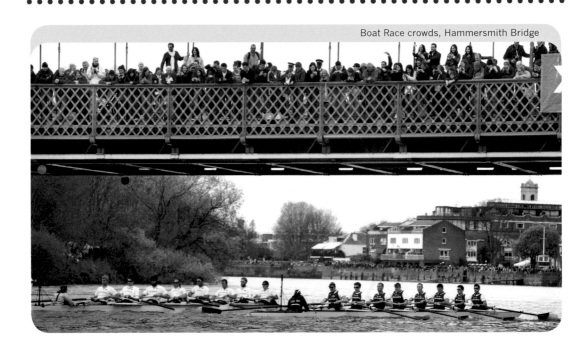

SPORTS DIARY OF THE YEAR

When these happen, the streets are noticeably quiet – until something exciting happens, when you hear the shouts and cheers coming out of people's windows!

FEBRUARY– MARCH:

Six Nations rugby

The Six Nations are England, France, Ireland, Italy, Scotland and Wales. Watching it on TV is fun – but if you can get tickets it's even more exciting. If you can, go to a match on the final day: the top team is usually decided then, so these are nerve-shredding games for the fans.

MARCH OR APRIL:

The Boat Race

The top rowers of Oxford and Cambridge universities battle it out over 6.8 km of the River Thames. It's free to watch from the bank, though it might be hard to find a space. About 250,000 people turned up in 2013 – and millions more watched on TV.

APRIL:

Grand National

The UK's most popular horse race is so popular that the government decided the race has to be shown free, on a TV channel everyone can access. First held in 1839, the Grand National is today watched by over 500 million people, in 140 different countries.

MAY:

FA Cup final, football

See page 21 for more information about the FA Cup.

JUNE–JULY:

Wimbledon

The Wimbledon Championships is the biggest tennis tournament in the world, the one every player dreams of winning. If you can't afford courtside tickets, don't panic: the hillside at Aorangi Terrace has a giant screen showing the big matches live.

OTHER EVENTS TO LOOK OUT FOR

These sports events do not happen every year, but when they're on, sports fans get excited:

The Ashes (cricket tournament between England and Australia every two years)

The Ryder Cup (Europe v. USA golf contest, held every two years)

Commonwealth Games (athletics event every four years: hosted by the Scottish city of Glasgow in 2014)

SPORT

STREET SPORTS AND TRADITIONAL GAMES

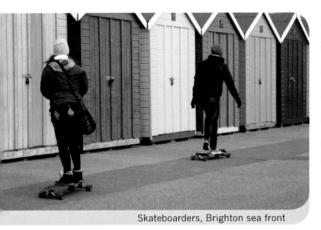

Skateboarders, Brighton sea front

Street sports and the UK's traditional games may not at first seem to have much in common. Both, though, often have an anarchic, slightly disorganised character. The lack of rules, regulations and referees is especially appealing to the UK's young people.

STREET SPORTS

Since most people in the UK live in cities, the appeal of sports you can do in any kind of urban environment is obvious.

Skateboarding
Most towns and cities have a skate park of some sort, and taking your skateboard to the local park is a good way to meet people.

BMX
BMX is one of the UK's most popular street sports, and some of the world's best riders are British: riders such as Danny MacAskill, Mike Mullen and Bas Keep.

Parkour/free running
Ever since the Bond film *Casino Royale* opened with a breathtaking parkour sequence, the activity of moving yourself forward using any object around you has become increasingly popular in the UK. Towns and cities with active parkour scenes include Glasgow, Manchester, Nottingham, Norwich, Aberystwyth, London and Exeter.

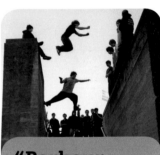

"Parkour is getting over all the obstacles in your path as you would in an emergency situation."

— David Belle, one of the founders of parkour

TRADITIONAL GAMES

Traditional games from hundreds of years ago are still popular in the UK. Here are three:

The Ba Game (Scotland)

The Ba Game is a kind of rugby-football mash-up played between large groups. It can be hours before a goal (which wins the contest) is scored.

Tug-of-war

Two teams take hold of opposite ends of a rope. Each tries to pull the other forward. Put a river or stream between them, and it gets really interesting.

Cheese rolling (Gloucestershire)

People carrying large, round cheeses climb a steep hill. Then they roll their cheese down, following behind as fast as possible. First cheese and person to the bottom wins. Unsurprisingly the event is known for injuries to those taking part (and even the spectators), with sprains and broken bones being common.

SPORT

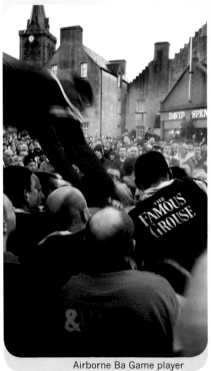

Airborne Ba Game player

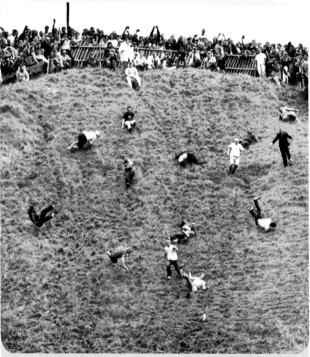

Cheese rollers in action

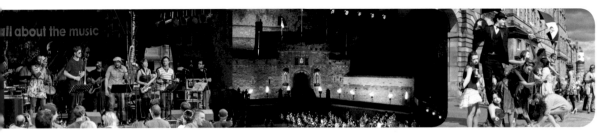

MUSIC

From rap to dance, pop, and folk, the UK has a thriving music scene. New bands spring up and disappear all the time. Most big towns have venues where you can see live music, ranging from small rooms that will hold 40 or 50 people to giant stadiums.

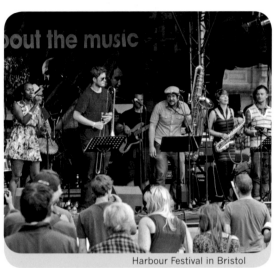

Harbour Festival in Bristol

THE BRITISH MUSIC EXPERIENCE

The British Music Experience in Greenwich, London is a great place to visit if you're into music. The museum has a rolling programme of exhibits about British music since 1945. You can see photos and videos of top bands, walk along the Sound Tunnel, gawp at old Spice Girls outfits, flick through the virtual collection of 12" singles in the Hey DJ! experience, and much more.

MUSIC FROM AROUND THE WORLD

The UK has been welcoming immigrants for centuries, and the new arrivals brought their music with them. As a result you can hear just about any kind of music imaginable on the UK's streets, from calypso to choral singing, didgeridoo playing, drumming and ukulele music.

MUSIC TO LISTEN OUT FOR

What are you most likely to hear coming from radios, being played in cafés, or live on stage in the UK? The most popular types of music include:

Rock:
the biggest UK bands include Coldplay and the wonderfully named British Sea Power; Mumford & Sons are a huge folk rock band.

Pop:
dominated by female singers, including Adele and Jessie J.

R&B:
foreign acts such as Rihanna and Nicki Minaj get a lot of radio play.

Rap and hip-hop:
British talents include Dizzee Rascal and Tinie Tempah.

Dance:
Scotland's Calvin Harris and Frenchman David Guetta are among the top DJ/producers.

• •

> "I make music for the hips, not the head."
>
> — Norman Cook, a.k.a. top British DJ Fatboy Slim

THE X-FACTOR

If you are in the UK between September and December, expect to hear people talking about *The X-Factor*. This TV show is a music competition that aims to find the most promising new act each year. *The X Factor* has been wildly popular since it began in 2004.

CULTURE

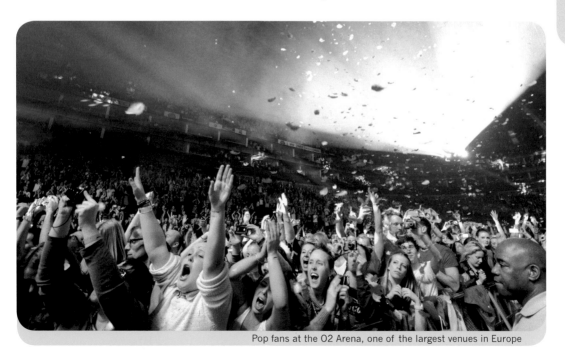

Pop fans at the O2 Arena, one of the largest venues in Europe

GLASTONBURY FESTIVAL

Glastonbury is Britain's biggest music festival, and one of the most famous in the world. This monster of an event happens almost every year, on the weekend in June closest to the longest day in the year. It is held on a farm in Somerset, in the south west of England.

Glastonbury is not a festival where you can turn up on the day and pay to get in. The 2013 event sold out all 135,000 tickets within two hours. If you ARE lucky enough to get a ticket, you'll hear all kinds of music inside the fence that surrounds the site, from rock to rap, R&B and dance.

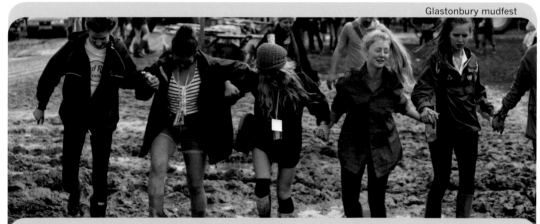
Glastonbury mudfest

GLASTONBURY SURVIVAL KIT CHECKLIST

There are a LOT of people at Glastonbury – and being the UK, it's quite likely to be rainy. What do you need to survive?

 Wellington boots
Wellies are the only way to keep your feet dry and clean if the ground gets muddy.

 Flag on a pole
Put this up beside your tent, so that you can find your tent among the thousands of other similar ones.

 Earplugs
Because even the biggest music fan has to sleep at some point!

OTHER MUSIC FESTIVALS

You could spend a very happy musical summer visiting festivals across the UK. There are over 300 each year. Here are four:

MAY:

Evolution
(Newcastle, England)

Held on three sites beside the River Tyne, Evolution is mostly dance and electronic music, with some hip-hop and pop.

JUNE:

Isle of Wight Festival
(Isle of Wight, England)

The grand old daddy of music festivals, this got so big and troublesome that in 1970 an Act of Parliament banned it! The festival restarted in 2002 and has been going ever since.

JULY:

T in the Park
(Kinross-shire, Scotland)

Rock, pop and dance all mixed together on a disused airfield outside the town of Kinross.

AUGUST:

Reading Festival
(Berkshire, England)

Mostly heavy metal, rock and pop, but with some dance and other music thrown in.

CULTURE

FOUNDING THE GLASTONBURY FESTIVAL

In 1970, a farmer and music fan called Michael Eavis decided to build a stage at his farm near Glastonbury, and invite bands to come and play. Everyone – festivalgoers and musicians – could camp in the fields. From the start Glastonbury attracted top acts: the first headliners were T-Rex, followed in 1971 by David Bowie.

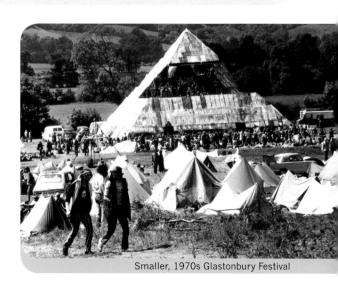

Smaller, 1970s Glastonbury Festival

EDINBURGH FESTIVAL

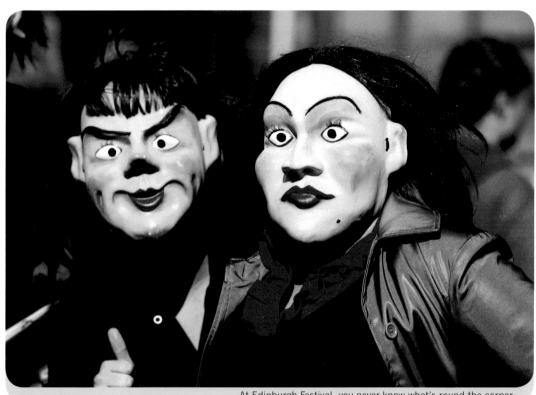

At Edinburgh Festival, you never know what's round the corner

The Edinburgh Fringe is said to be the biggest arts festival in the world. It specialises in comedy and theatre, but you can also see cutting-edge dance and music. In 2012, the Fringe lasted 25 days, during which there were 2,695 shows. Put another way, that's almost five shows an hour, every hour, all day and night.

WHAT TO SEE?

With so many performances, it can be a bit tricky to work out what you want to see. One good place for information is the pedestrian area around St Giles' Cathedral. Here, performers hand out flyers, and sometimes perform excerpts from their show as a taster.

"You know who really gives kids a bad name? Posh and Becks."

— unofficial best joke at the 2012 Edinburgh Festival, by comedian Stewart Francis

OTHER EDINBURGH FESTIVAL EVENTS

The Fringe is not the only festival based in Edinburgh. Here are three of the others (two of which also happen in August):

Edinburgh International Festival

This was started after the Second World War, to promote the 'flowering of the human spirit' after five years of conflict. It features classical music, theatre and dance: something to occupy your parents, perhaps?

Royal Edinburgh Military Tattoo

If you like the idea of sitting in an old castle watching marching bands and people dragging guns back and forth, the Military Tattoo is for you. It is so popular that it's said to be televised in 30 countries and is watched by 100 million people each year.

Edinburgh International Film Festival

The world's oldest continuously running film festival, EIFF used to happen in August alongside the rest of the Festival. It now takes place in June.

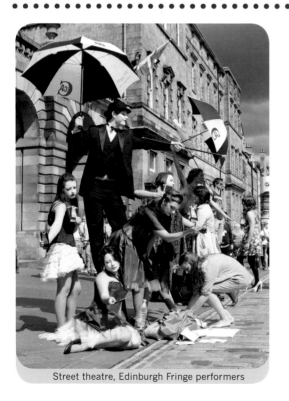

Street theatre, Edinburgh Fringe performers

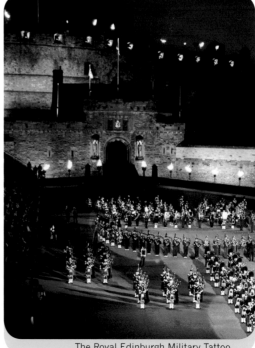

The Royal Edinburgh Military Tattoo

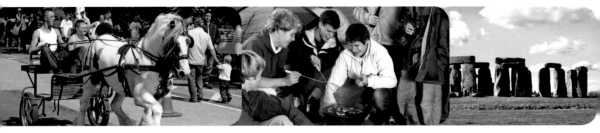

HOLIDAYS

The UK is a great place to take a holiday. It's so small that four days is long enough for a trip to almost anywhere. Whether you want cities, countryside, beaches or mountains, it's all within reach!

A VISIT TO THE SOUTHWEST

One of the most popular holidays in the UK is a visit to the southwest of England. Here are a few questions you'll need to ask yourself before your trip:

Beaches or moors?

Do you want to surf the Atlantic waves of the north coast? Or would you rather walk on the inland moors, hunting for ancient standing stones?

Camping or a roof over your head?

There are campsites everywhere (see pages 34–35). You can also stay in a teepee, a treehouse or a shiny-steel American caravan. If you prefer to sleep indoors, there are plenty of 'Bed and Breakfasts' (B&Bs) and hotels.

Self-catering or not?

During the summer, campsites are filled with the smell of barbecues. But if you don't want to cook your own food, try a take-away pasty – a pastry parcel filled with meat and vegetables.

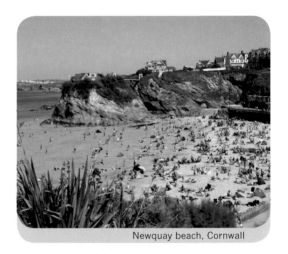
Newquay beach, Cornwall

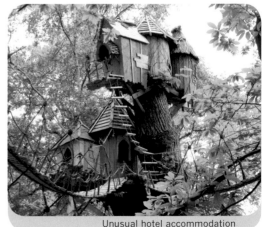
Unusual hotel accommodation

HOLIDAY HOTSPOTS IN THE UK

LAKE DISTRICT
First popular in the Victorian era, the Lakes (and the surrounding mountains) are still a favourite destination.

HIGHLANDS AND ISLANDS
Visit the UK's tallest mountains, then continue the adventure by ferry-hopping between islands off the coast.

YORKSHIRE DALES
Known for breathtaking walking and cycling routes on the hills, and pretty villages hidden in the valleys.

NORTHERN IRELAND BEACHES
A well-kept secret, these are popular with surfers, walkers and (when possible) sunbathers.

THE BROADS
A boating holiday destination, the area also attracts ramblers, artists, anglers and bird-watchers.

SOUTHWEST WALES
The Gower Peninsula and Pembrokeshire each have beautiful sandy beaches and countryside.

SOUTHWEST ENGLAND
Also called the West Country – see **Visit to the southwest** on page 32 for details.

LEISURE

CAMPING BRITAIN

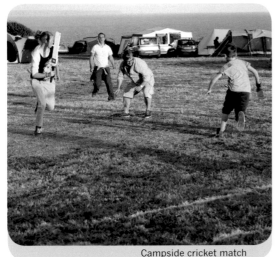

Campside cricket match

In the last 10 years the number of campers in the UK has grown massively. Some go camping for a weekend away from the city, others for a family holiday near the beach. Whatever the reason, the UK's campsites have never been busier.

WHERE CAN YOU CAMP?

In England, Wales and Northern Ireland, you are only really allowed to camp on an official campsite. These range from big sites with swimming pools, entertainment centres and laundries, to farmers' fields with a toilet in the corner. Some even offer 'glamping' (short for 'glamorous camping').

In Scotland, things are different. You can camp practically anywhere! The only rules for 'wild camping' are:

- Avoid farmland, whether for animals or crops

- Camp well away from buildings, ancient monuments and roads

- Don't stay more than three nights in one place

- Take your rubbish away with you

- Leave the camping spot as you found it

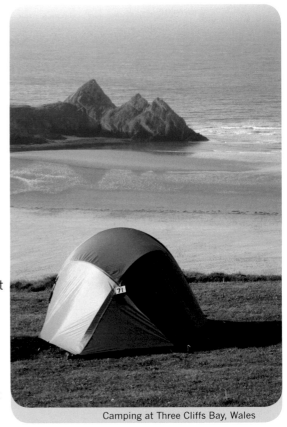

Camping at Three Cliffs Bay, Wales

ART OF THE BARBECUE: 3 STEPS TO BARBECUE HEAVEN.

1. Place your barbecue on something that a) doesn't wobble and b) won't catch light.

2. Use firelighters and wait until the coals are white before putting on your food.

3. Check that the food is cooked right through before you eat it.

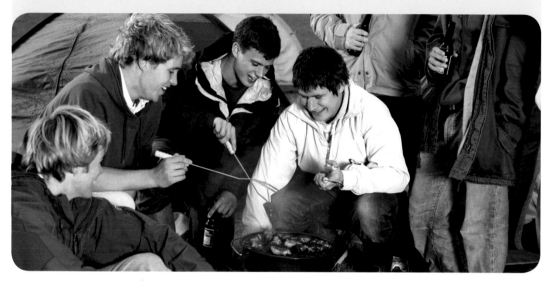

CAMPING SURVIVAL CHECKLIST

Camping is great fun as long as you're warm, dry and comfortable. This checklist will make sure you are!

 Tent
A tent with an inner and outer layer is best. Pitch your tent on level ground and peg it out so that the sides don't flap.

Sleeping bag
Pick a 2-season bag for warm weather, a 3- or 4-season if it's colder.

 Sleep mat and pillow
Having these will make sure you have a good night's sleep.

 Hat and fleece
If you get cold at night, putting on a hat is a great way to warm up.

 Wellies or flip-flops
Shoes you can take on and off quickly before getting in the tent.

COUNTRY FAIRS

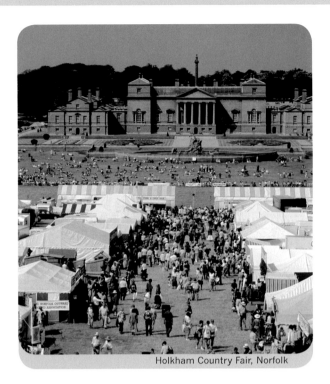

Holkham Country Fair, Norfolk

If there's one event that is typically British, it's a summer fair. Many of these are enormous, with funfairs and row after row of stalls selling products and all sorts of food. In fact, you might find it hard to believe that some fairs are hundreds of years old.

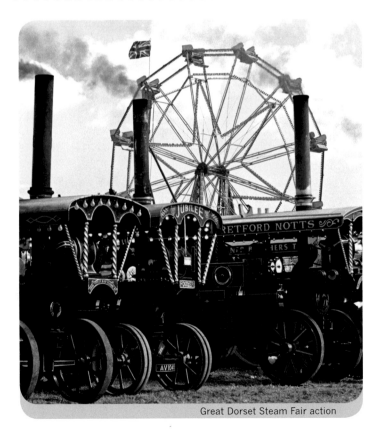

Great Dorset Steam Fair action

THE GREAT DORSET STEAM FAIR

If you are interested in steam-powered anything, head for north Dorset in August. The Great Dorset Steam Fair's most popular attractions include tractors, traction engines and farm machinery. But there's also a steam-powered funfair, classic cars and motorbikes, and working heavy horses to see. Just be sure to leave plenty of time for your journey. The roads will be clogged with owners driving their steam-powered vehicles to and from the show. Some of these only do about 15 kph, so they can be overtaken on a bicycle!

ON THE MENU AT THE FAIR

If you stumble on a small village fair, there will almost certainly be a choice of traditional fair-time food. Take your pick from:

- Sponge cakes
- Cucumber or cheese-and-tomato sandwiches
- Tea or lemonade

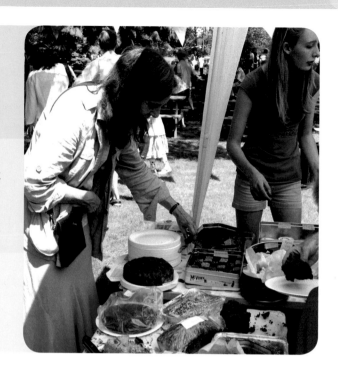

OTHER OUTDOOR EVENTS

The Great Dorset Steam Fair may be the biggest, but it's not the only outdoor event. Here are two more oddball choices:

Appleby Horse Fair
(Cumbria, England)

Since 1685, Gypsies from across the British Isles have been coming to Appleby. They head here every June, to buy and sell horses and to meet with relatives and friends. There is a similar fair eight weeks later in Brough, Cumbria.

Whitstable Oyster Festival
(Kent, England)

There has been an oyster festival in Whitstable ever since the Romans started tucking into the local shellfish. It takes place every July. If you don't like oysters, look out for the belly-dancing lessons and Blessing of the Sea ceremony.

LEISURE

Trotting through the streets of Appleby

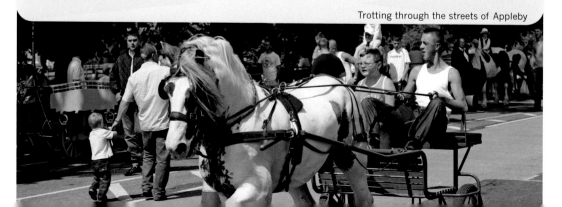

VISIT ANCIENT BRITAIN

The UK is littered with traces of the ancient peoples who lived there thousands of years ago. They are most common in the western regions: England's southwest, Wales, western Scotland and Northern Ireland. These places were occupied tens of thousands of years ago by Celtic tribes.

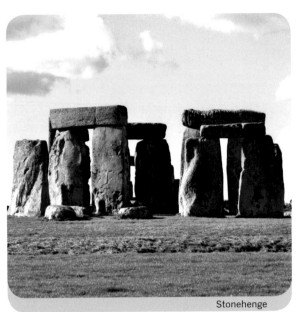
Stonehenge

STONE CIRCLES TO VISIT

Arriving at either of these lonely places at dawn or sunset makes it easy to imagine what they must have been like thousands of years ago:

Stonehenge, Wiltshire, England

The UK's most famous stone circle is on Salisbury Plain, a high, flat area of land that stretches into the distance.

Callanish, Isle of Lewis, Scotland

A local legend says that these stones are the remains of giants, who were turned to stone as a punishment for not becoming Christians – however, the stones pre-date Christianity.

STONE CIRCLES AND STANDING STONES

There are hundreds of ancient standing stones in the UK, many of them visible from a car or train window. Some are arranged into stone circles, while others stand alone, often on lonely hilltops. Many circles are associated with strange legends. The Merry Maidens in Cornwall are said to be the remnants of local girls turned to stone for dancing on a Sunday. One of the giant stones at Avebury in Wiltshire is said to cross the road at midnight. And chipping bits off the Rollright Stones apparently brings down a deadly curse on your head.

HILL FORTS

There are ancient hill forts, where ancient people cut terraces into the hillsides and built defences, all around the UK. There are over 3,000 in total. You're most likely to see them in southwest England, the west coasts of Wales and Scotland, and in the border areas between England, Scotland and Wales. Walking up to one of these and imagining yourself as someone from the ancient world is a great way to spend an hour or two.

HILL FORTS TO VISIT

Pen Dynas, Ceredigion, Wales

Overlooking the sea, and with rivers on two sides, Pen Dynas is one of the biggest hill forts in Wales.

Yeavering Bell, Northumberland, England

This would have been a hill fort with a difference, because its walls are made of a local stone that starts life pink! These days the colour has faded to dull grey.

Maiden Castle, Dorset, England

Among the largest and most complex of Iron Age hill forts in Europe.

THE CULT OF MITHRAS

The Romans brought the Cult of Mithras to Britain. Little is known about the Cult, but it was associated with the military. We know that members met in caverns or underground halls, and sacrificed bulls to the god. Secret Roman temples of Mithras have been discovered underground. At Temple Court, London, one of these is open to visitors.

Maiden Castle Iron Age hill fort, Dorchester, Dorset

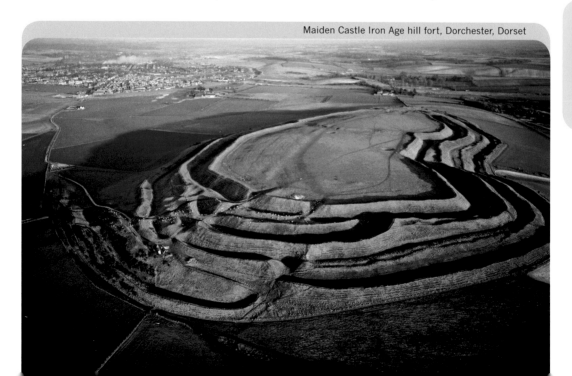

LEISURE

NORTHERN **IRELAND**

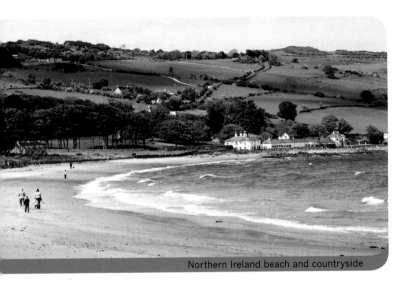
Northern Ireland beach and countryside

Northern Ireland is the only part of the UK that isn't on the island of Great Britain. Instead, it shares the island of Ireland with the Republic of Ireland. It is an increasingly popular place to visit.

PROTESTANT AND CATHOLIC

Northern Ireland has two main communities, based on people's religion. The first is the Protestants, who mostly think it is important for Northern Ireland to be part of the UK. The second community is the Catholics, many of whom think Northern Ireland ought to be part of the Republic of Ireland. In the past, arguments over this subject have become violent.

Until recently, this violence has kept visitors away. These days the communities live more peacefully and more visitors come to the area. Northern Ireland's key attractions are its scenery, heritage and sporting activities.

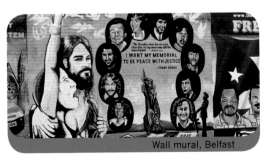
Wall mural, Belfast

1922: THE DIVISION OF IRELAND

For generations before 1922, the island of Ireland was part of the UK. After years of protests by Irish people, most of the island became an independent country in 1922. Only the northeast corner was kept as part of the UK.

THE *CRAIC*

In Ireland you often hear people talking about 'the *craic*' (pronounced 'crack'). There's no direct translation for this word, but it means a good time, something that's a lot of fun.

TOP ATTRACTIONS

This insider guide will give you some ideas for a visit to Northern Ireland:

Walk on the Giant's Causeway

Thousands of rock pillars, which look as if they have been carved, are actually the result of an ancient volcanic eruption.

Hide yourself away at Binders Cove

Over a thousand years ago, this underground passageway was built to hide people and treasures from Viking raiders.

Take a black-taxi tour of Belfast

Black cabs are a traditional way to get around, and some offer tours of the city. Keep a special eye out for Belfast's colourful wall murals.

Check out St George's Market, Belfast

This old covered market is somewhere to pick up anything from buttons to shoes, lampshades or even shark meat.

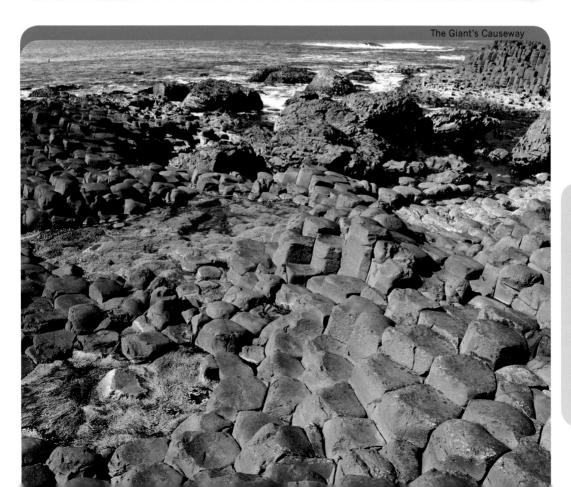
The Giant's Causeway

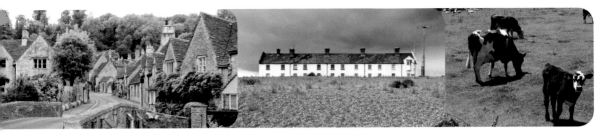

KEY INFORMATION
FOR TRAVELLERS

LANGUAGE

English is spoken everywhere. The Welsh language had almost disappeared by the 1980s, but has been brought back to life and is now widely spoken in Wales. In Scotland and Northern Ireland, Gaelic is sometimes spoken.

ENTERING THE UK

People from European Union countries can enter the UK without a visa, though arrivals at airports and ferry ports usually have to show their passport.

Visitors from other countries may need a visa, so it is important to check with your own government whether this is required.

GETTING AROUND

The UK has a good railway system connecting its cities and towns, though trains can be expensive unless tickets are booked in advance (see www.nationalrail. co.uk). Buses run in large cities and towns, though in rural areas they may not appear often, if at all. Cycling is a good way to travel short distances, but only folding bikes can be taken on busy trains.

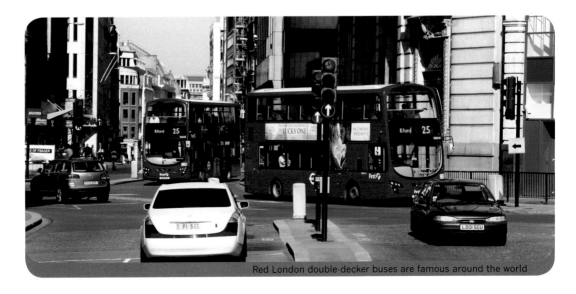

Red London double-decker buses are famous around the world

HEALTH

If you have a minor health problem such as a sore throat, a pharmacy could be a good source of help.

Almost everyone who needs to see a doctor in Britain uses the National Health Service. Emergency treatment is free, but visitors from other countries usually have to pay for non-emergency medical help.

POSTAL SERVICES

The main postal service in the UK is provided by the Post Office. You can buy stamps at post offices and at many other shops: newsagents are a likely place to buy them.

Letters can be posted in the red post boxes that are a common sight on street corners. Parcels have to be taken to a post office for posting. Use first class mail for urgent post as second class mail takes a few days. International mail will take even longer.

MOBILE NETWORKS

The main European mobile-phone networks are all available in the UK. Using a foreign phone – even on the same network as you have at home – is expensive, especially for data, so it's important to turn off data roaming unless you have a UK SIM card. (If you are visiting the UK for a long time, it is easy and inexpensive to buy a SIM with a monthly unlimited-data payment.)

INTERNET PROVISION

The UK generally has excellent Internet provision. Free wifi zones are available in many public spaces, hotels and cafés. Cybercafés offer paid Internet access and computer use, and public libraries often offer the same thing free or for a small charge.

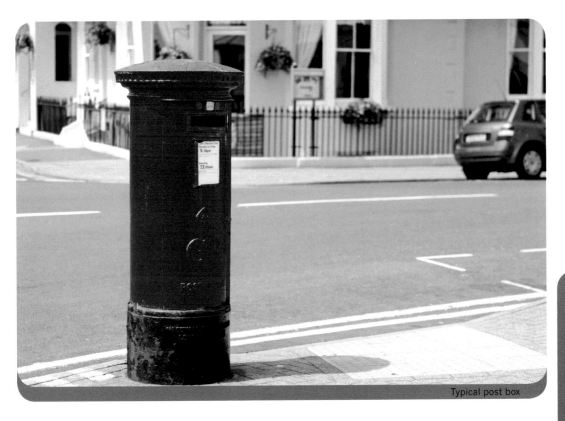

Typical post box

CURRENCY:

Pound (£1 = roughly €1.18, or $1.5). Currency exchange is available at larger banks, bureau de change, post offices, some department stores and train stations.

TIME ZONE:

Greenwich Mean Time (GMT)

On the last Sunday in March, the UK switches to British Summer Time and clocks are put forward one hour. On the last Sunday in October clocks are put back to GMT.

TELEPHONE DIALLING CODES:

To call the UK from outside the country, add 44 to the beginning of the number, and drop the zero.

To call another country from the UK, add OO and the country code of the place you are dialling to the beginning of the number, and drop the zero.

OPENING HOURS:

In cities and towns, most shops are open by 10:00 and closed by 19:00 from Monday to Saturday. On Sundays, they are usually open between 11:00 and 16:00. Some shops open for much longer, for example from 07:00 to 23:00, and a few stay open 24 hours a day, 7 days a week.

In the countryside, shops are generally open 09:00–18:00, but may be closed on Saturday and Wednesday afternoons, and all day on Sunday.

DECIPHERING ENGLISH:

British people don't always mean what they seem to mean – in fact, sometimes they mean the opposite. Here are a few English phrases that can trip up visitors:

English person says:	Visitor hears:	Actual meaning:
Quite good.	Quite good.	Not very good.
It's probably my fault...	He thinks it's his fault.	It's not my fault. It's yours.
With respect...	I respect you.	I have no respect for you.
Of course, you do have other options.	You have a choice.	Your current choice is stupid.

FINDING OUT MORE

BOOKS TO READ: NON-FICTION

The Smell of Poo Closed Parliament! The Fact or Fiction behind London Adam Sutherland (Wayland, 2012)
Part of an excellent series exploring the truth (or otherwise) behind common myths, this is a great, fun-filled read about London. There's a second history title called *Medieval People Washed Their Clothes In Wee* by Kay Barnham.

London: A Time Traveller's Guide Moira Butterfield (Franklin Watts, 2013)
Imagine you could step into a time machine and travel through the centuries to discover some of London's hidden secrets. This book takes you on an incredible trip through London's amazing story.

BOOKS TO READ: FICTION

Goodnight Mr Tom Michelle Margorian
When Willie Beech is evacuated to the countryside during the Second World War, he is a sad, damaged boy. But Willie slowly works his way to a better place with the help of his host, old Tom Oakley.

Stoneheart Trilogy Charlie Fletcher (Hodder)
The trilogy, set in the streets of London, follows George and Edie, as they struggle to repair the damage George has done at the start of the story by breaking a stone dragon statue.

The Story of Tracey Beaker Jacqueline Wilson
The 'autobiography' of Tracey Beaker, rebel and resident of The Dumping Ground – a children's home from which Tracey dreams of one day being rescued by her glamorous mother.

WEBSITES

http://www.visitbritain.com
This is a government-backed site. It is aimed not only at people who want to visit Britain, but also British people who would like to see a new part of the country. It is packed with information, but the most useful sections are probably 'Things to do' and 'Destinations and maps'.

There are individual sites for each of the four areas that make up the UK:
www.visitengland.org,
www.visitscotland.co.uk,
www.visitwales.com
www.discovernorthernireland.com.

https://www.cia.gov/library/publications/the-world-factbook/geos/uk.html
This link will take you to the CIA (Central Intelligence Agency) web page about the United Kingdom. It's quite dry, but crammed full of useful information and statistics.

Note to parents and teachers:
Every effort has been made by the Publishers to ensure that these websites are suitable for children, that they are of the highest educational value, and that they contain no inappropriate or offensive material. However, because of the nature of the Internet, it is impossible to guarantee that the contents of these sites will not be altered. We strongly advise that Internet access is supervised by a responsible adult.

THE ESSENTIALS

INDEX